Pediatric Nursing Procedures

Second Edition

Raman Kalia MSc (N)
Gold Medalist
Punjab University Chandigarh, India
PhD (Pediatric Surgery), PGI Chandigarh, India

Presently
Director-Principal, Saraswati Nursing Institute
Dhianpura, Kurali, Distt. Ropar
Punjab, India

Formerly
Lecturer, National Institute of
Nursing Education (PGIMER)
Chandigarh, India

Foreword
Indarjit Walia

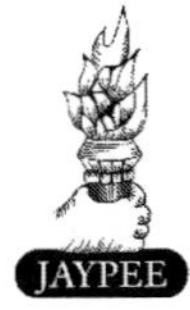

JAYPEE BROTHERS MEDICAL PUBLISHERS
The Health Sciences Publisher
New Delhi | London

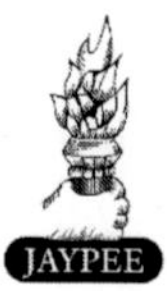

Jaypee Brothers Medical Publishers (P) Ltd

Headquarters
EMCA House, 23/23-B Ansari Road,
Daryaganj New Delhi 110 002, India
Landline: +91-11-23272143,
+91-11-23272703
+91-11-23282021, +91-11-23245672
e-mail: jaypee@jaypeebrothers.com

Corporate Office
4838/24, Ansari Road,
Daryaganj New Delhi 110 002, India
Phone: +91-11-43574357
Fax: +91-11-43574314
e-mail: jaypee@jaypeebrothers.com

Overseas Office
JP Medical Ltd.
83, Victoria Street, London
SW1H 0HW (UK)
Phone: +44-20 3170 8910
e-mail: info@jpmedpub.com

EU GPSR Authorised Representative
Logos Europe, 9 rue Nicolas Poussin
17000, La Rochelle, France
Phone: +33 (0) 6 67 93 73 78
e-mail: contact@logoseurope.eu

Website: www.jaypeebrothers.com
Website: www.jaypeedigital.com

Inquiries for bulk sales may be solicited at: jaypee@jaypeebrothers.com

Pediatric Nursing Procedures
First Edition: 2012
Second Edition: 2015
Reprint: 2026
ISBN 978-93-5152-623-0
Printed at: Samrat Offset Pvt. Ltd.

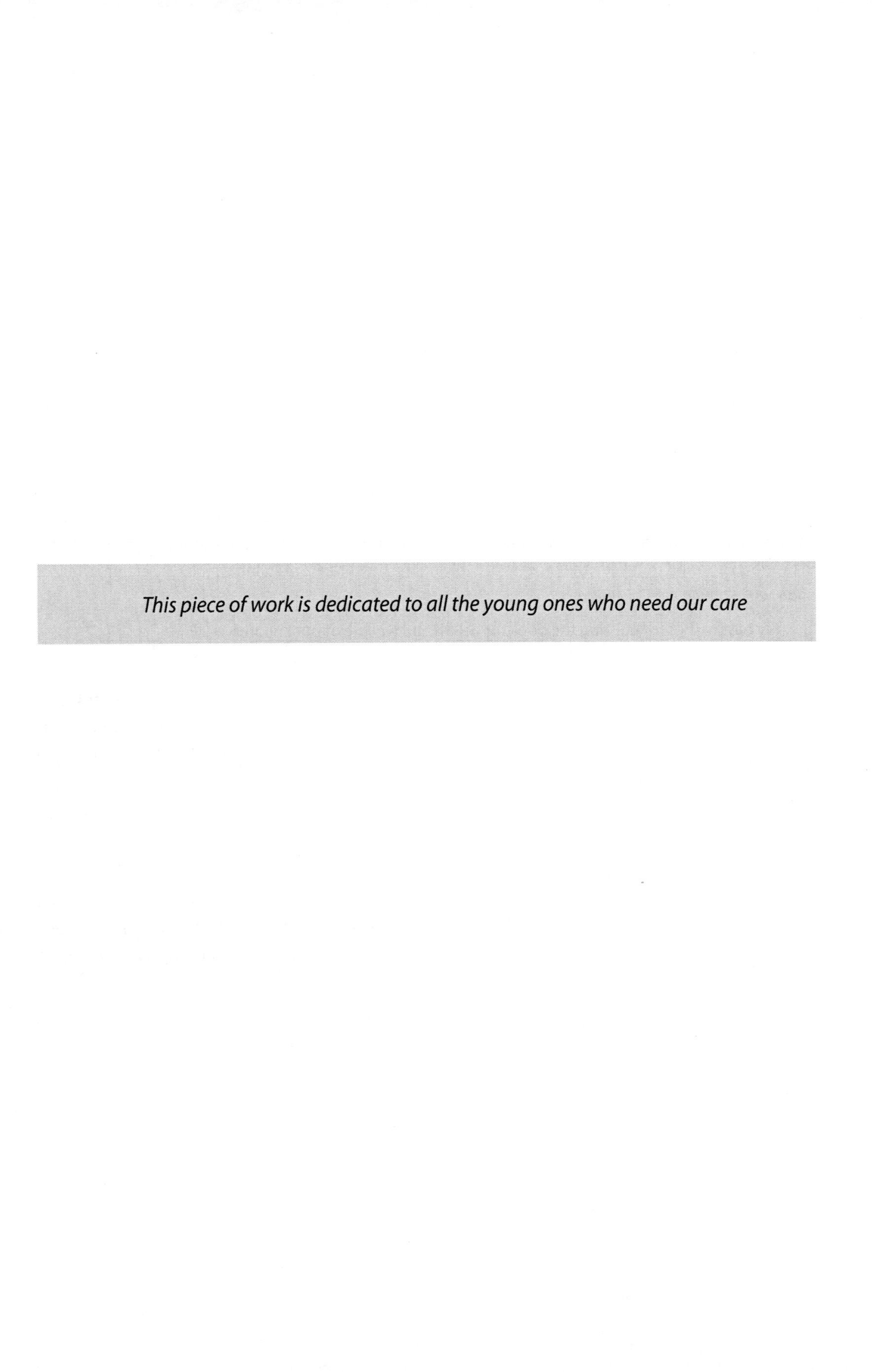

This piece of work is dedicated to all the young ones who need our care

Foreword

Literature on nursing procedures especially for sick children is rare and inadequate for use in Indian health institutions. Nurses acquire competency by practicing on instructions from senior nurses/nursing teachers. Whereas written document on steps of performing nursing task would be safe and valid. Written document would help setting standard of pediatric nursing practice, and shall be helpful for nursing teachers to demonstrate the correct process of care of children.

I am so very satisfied with the attempt of the author of this book to provide practical resource material for students, teachers and practical nurses. I am sure this ready material would set nurses critically analyze each set of procedure as per their institute policy and facilities, convey it to the author for incorporating it in the next issue and thus keep the process of evolving the best literature suitable for large section of nurses engaged in taking care of children.

My best wishes for utilizing the book for health and welfare of our children.

Indarjit Walia
Teacher and Community
Health Nursing Practitioner

Presently
Consultant and Professor
Rattan Group of Institutes, Sohana
Mohali, Punjab, India

Formerly
Principal, National Institute of Nursing Education
PGIMER Chandigarh, India

Preface

Nursing students and staff need to have competency in performing *Pediatric Nursing Procedures* while delivering child health services. Indian nursing council have recommended set pediatric nursing procedures to be competently demonstrated to the students and get return demonstration for certifying them as qualified to register as nurses with the nursing council. Health institutions expect nurses to perform pediatric care as per set norms in the form of procedures. Whereas nursing literature is short of steps of procedures to be performed for looking after sick children in Indian health institutions. Hence, this book on pediatric nursing procedures is a step toward filling gap in the required literatures.

The book is learner-friendly, divided in two sections. The first section is on basic nursing procedures and second section is on advanced nursing procedures. Each procedure is covered under subheadings, e.g. introduction, definition, purpose, methods, articles required and steps of procedures. Explanation whereever required and special points to remember while performing procedure are added for the benefit of the readers. Some useful text is arranged in the appendices at the end of the book.

It gives me immense pleasure while preparing the second edition of the book, I am grateful to the reviewers for giving suggestions and thus providing me guidelines for adding advanced nursing procedures of neonatal care and intensive care of babies. I also thank the readers for accepting and appreciating the contents of the procedures. However the real nursing care is incorporating the theory into practice.

This book shall be useful for all beginners in pediatric nursing whether a general nurse midwife, BSc nurse, or postgraduate nurses . A set of this book in each pediatric ward shall be of immense help.

Raman Kalia

Acknowledgments

A little effort like this is possible only due to the blessings of Almighty. I would like to express my gratitude to Dr Indarjit Walia, Ex-Principal NINE, PGIMER Chandigarh, for constant guidance and encouragement during the professional academic ventures. A word of thanks to all the colleagues for their contribution and critical analysis of the book. I express gratitude to Mrs Amiteshwar (MSc N Child Health Nursing) Ms Ruchi (Msc N Staff Nurse, Paediatric ICU PGIMER) for contributing towards restructuring of the contents of the Second Edition of the book.

The author wishes to acknowledge the contribution of M/s Jaypee Brothers Medical Publishers (P) Ltd, New Delhi, India for typing the manuscript and finally shaping it in its present form.

I am also indebted to my family, husband and children Tushar and Arushi for allowing me to spare time for this work.

Contents

SECTION 1 BASIC NURSING PROCEDURES

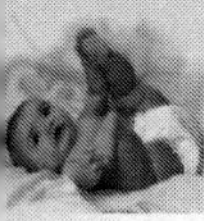

SECTION 2 ADVANCED NURSING PROCEDURES

SECTION

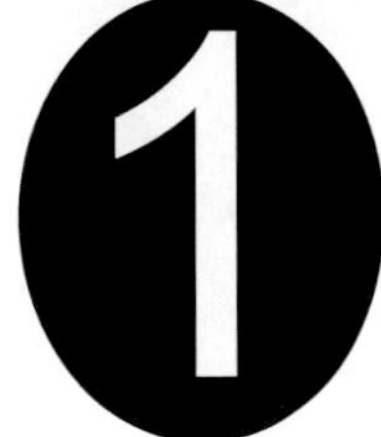

Basic Nursing Procedures

CHAPTER

Physical Assessment

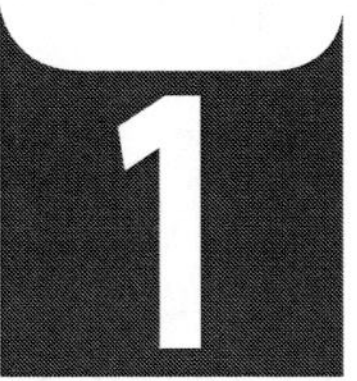

Introduction

Once an infant is born he/she requires a thorough skilled observation and examination to ensure a satisfactory adjustment to the extrauterine life. The physical assessment represents a screening procedure to identify the likelihood of any pathology in a specific system to identify any deviation or abnormality in that system.

During physical assessment it is essential that the infant should not be disturbed so that a successful examination can be conducted.

Definition

It is a thorough inspection or a detailed study of the entire body or some part of the body to determine the general physical or mental conditions of the body.

Purpose

- To understand the physical and mental well-being of the patient.
- To detect disease in its early stage.
- To determine the cause and the extent of disease.
- To understand any changes in the condition of disease, any improvement or regression.
- To determine the nature of the treatment or nursing care needed for the patient.
- To safeguard the patient and his family by noting the early signs.
- To contribute to the medical research.

Methods

Inspection

- Visual examination of the body is called inspection.

Palpation

- It is the feeling of the body or a part with the hands to note the size and positions of the organs.

Percussion

- It is the examination by tapping with the fingers on the body to determine the condition of the internal organs by the sound that are produced.

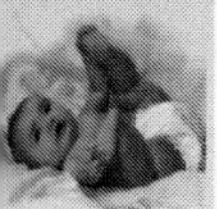

Auscultation

- It is the listening to sound within the body with the aid of the stethoscope.

Manipulation

- It is the moving of a part of the body to note its flexibility.

Testing of reflexes

- Testing reflexes is an important part of the neurological examination.

Articles Required

- Stethoscope.
- TPR Tray.
- Tape measure.
- Torch.
- Weighing machine.
- Paper and pen.
- Draw sheet.
- Scale.

Preparation of Patient and Environment

Patient

If the child is old enough, explain procedure to the patient to gain cooperation if not, then explain to parents.

Environment

- Maintenance of privacy.
- Proper lighting.
- Comfortable bed.

Steps of the Procedure

1. **General appearance**
   - *Nourishment:* Well-nourished or undernourished.
   - *Body build:* Thin or obese.
   - *Health:* Healthy or unhealthy.
   - *Activity:* Active or dull.
2. **Mental status**
   - *Consciousness:* Conscious, unconscious, delirious.
   - *Look:* Anxious, worried, depressed.

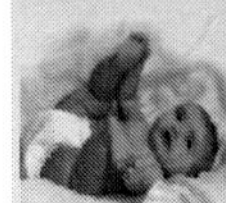

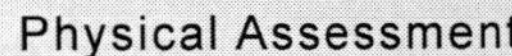

3. **Posture**
   - *Body Curves:* Lordosis, kyphosis, scoliosis.
   - *Movement:* Any limp.

Vital Signs

First take respiration count, then count heart rate, at the end temperature is recorded. In this sequence examiner will be able to count respiratory rate and heart rate without disturbing the child. Place the thermometer parallel to the body in axilla.

Normal Range in Newborn Baby

- **Temperature:** 36.5 to 37.5°C.
- **Heart rate:** 120 to 160 beats/min.
- **Respiratory rate:** 40 to 60 breaths/min.
- **BP:** 25/40 to 45/60 mm of Hg.

Height

- **In infants:** Spread the draw sheet on hard surface and place the baby over it. Straighten the lower extremities. With the help of scale, mark the markings at head and foot end. Measure the height with measuring tape in centimeters.
- **In children:** Make the child stand against the wall so that his head, shoulders, buttocks and heels touch the wall. Mark the height and measure it.

  Normal height in Newborn Baby: 48 to 53 cm.

Weight

Normal weight of New Born Baby: 2.5 to 3.5 Kg.

Skin Conditions

- **Color:** Pallor, jaundice, cyanosis, flushing.
- **Texture:** Dryness, flaking, wrinkling or excessive moisture.
- **Temperature:** Warm, cold, clammy.
- **Lesions:** Macules, papules, vesicles, wounds.

Head and Face

Shape of skull and fontanels. Anterior fontanels closes at 18 months and posterior fontanels at 1 and a half months. Check fontanels are flat elevated or depressed.

- **Skull circumference in newborn:** 33 to 38 cm.
- **Scalp:** Cleanliness, hair, dandruff, pediculi, cephalohematoma.
- **Face:** Pale, flushed, puffiness, fatigue, pain, fear, anxiety.

  Eye: Assess for pale conjunctiva, jaundiced sclera, reaction of pupils to light, discharge, redness, squint.

  Ear: Assess for crusts or discharge, deviated nasal septum.

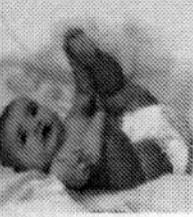

Mouth and Pharynx

- **Lips:** Redness, swelling, crusts, cyanosis, stomatitis.
- **Odor of mouth:** Foul smelling.
- **Teeth:** Discolouration and dental caries.
- **Mucus membrane and gums:** Ulceration, bleeding, swelling.
- **Tongue:** Pale, dry lesions, tongue ties.
- **Throat and Pharynx:** Enlarged tonsils, redness and pus.

Neck

- **Lymph Nodes:** Enlarged, palpable.
- **Thyroid gland:** Enlarged.
- **Range of motion:** Flexion, extension and rotation.
- **Rashes:** in Skin Folds in Newborn Baby.

Chest

Assess for shape of thorax, breath sounds, sometimes discharge from the nipples of new born girl is present due to maternal hormone, normal chest circumference in new born is 30 to 35 cm.

Abdomen

- **Observation:** Redness around umbilical cord, rashes, scar, hernia, ascites, distension.
- **Auscultation:** Bowel sounds.
- **Palpation:** Liver margin, palpable spleen, inguinal hernia.
- **Percussion:** Presence of gas, fluid or masses.
- Normal Abdomen Circumference in newborn baby is 29 to 32 cm.

Extremities

Assess for joints, tremors, clubbing of fingers, polydactyly, syndactyly.

Back

Assess for spinal bifida, curves.

Genitals and Rectum

Assess testis has descended into scrotum, pseudomensuration, inguinal lymph nodes, patency of urinary meatus and rectum, frequency of urine and stool per day.

Reflexes

- **Eye:** Blinking, pupillary, doll.
- **Nose:** Sneeze, gladbellar.
- **Mouth and Throat:** Sucking, gag, rooting.
- **Extremities:** Grasp, babinski.
- **Mass:** Moro, startle, dance.

CHAPTER 2

Measurement of Weight, Length and Height

Definition

It is procedure carried out to find out weight of a child.

Purpose

- To estimate normal growth and development of the child.
- To facilitate calculation of drug according to weight of the child.

Points to Remember

Inspection

- Balance the scale by setting it at zero before, checking the weight.
- Measure the weight in a comfortable warm room.
- Weigh the infants and toddlers nude.
- Older children are usually weighed while wearing their under pants or light clothing. However, you should respect the privacy of all children.
- Weight should be checked everyday at the same time and usually before the feed (especially in case of premature babies).
- Weight should be checked with the same scale daily.

Articles Required

- Weighing scale on a trolley or table.
- Small towel or diaper to cover the scale basket.
- Patient's Chart.

Steps of the Procedure

1. Explain the procedure to mother.
2. Place Small towel or diaper to cover the scale basket.
3. Place the baby on the basket.

After Care

- Record the weight on the chart and compare it with the normal.

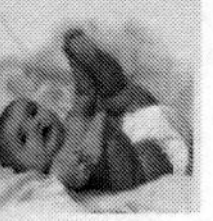

- If the child is wearing some types of special device such as splints or prosthesis you must note this while recording weight.
- Clean the weighing scale with antiseptic lotion.
- Dry the scale and replace it in its correct place.

LENGTH

Definition

Length refer to measurement of the body from head to toe before the age of 3 years to avoid postural errors in supine position with the help of infantometer, i.e. horizontal board with fixed head moving foot end.

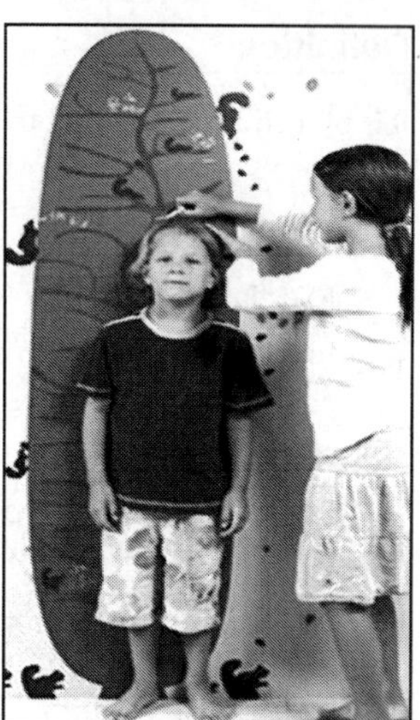

Purpose

To estimate normal growth and development of the child.

Points to Remember

The heal board should be vertical and knees should be hold straight.

Articles Required

- Infantometer on a trolley or table.
- Small towel or diaper to cover the scale basket
- Patient's chart.

Steps of the Procedure

1. Explain the procedure to mother.
2. Wash your hands.
3. Remove the clothes of the infant.
4. Lift the infant gently from his crib/bed and place him on the infantometer.
5. Place the head firmly at the top of the board and the heels against the foot board.
6. Note the length of the baby.

HEIGHT

Definition

Measurement from head to toe with the help of stadiometer after the age of three years.

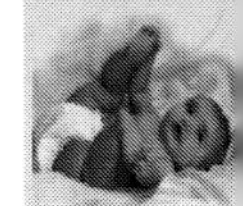

Steps of the Procedure

1. Explain the procedure to the mother.
2. Measure height by having child stand as tall and straight as possible with the head in midline.
3. Be sure that child's back is towards the vertical flat with the heels, buttocks and back of shoulders touching the flat surface.
4. A horizontal head board is lowered up to the head while subject inhales and reading is taken at eye level.

After Care

- Record the length/height on the chart and compare it with the normal for the age.
- Replace the infantometer and stadiometer.

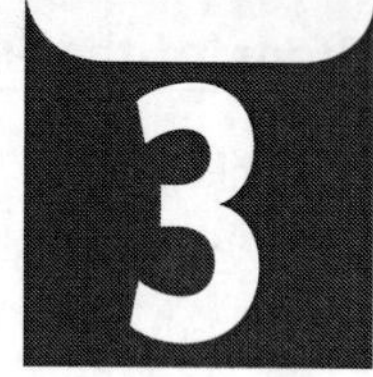

Recording Vital Signs

Introduction

Vital signs provide clues to the severity of the disease and early signs of complications. These needs to be carefully measured and any deviations are reported and recorded. The volume and character of urine are noted and the child is weighed daily.

Definition

Temperature, heart rate, respiration and blood pressure are known as vital signs because these are governed by vital organs.

Normal Vital Signs in Children

Normal vital signs in childhood

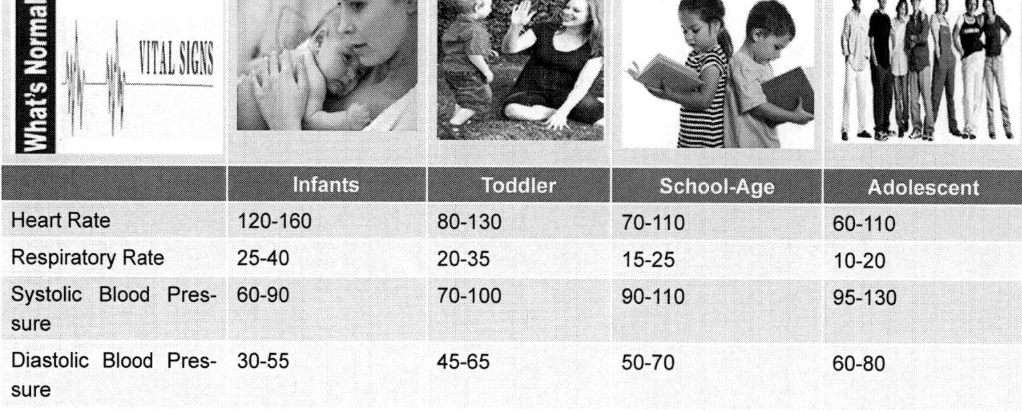

	Infants	Toddler	School-Age	Adolescent
Heart Rate	120-160	80-130	70-110	60-110
Respiratory Rate	25-40	20-35	15-25	10-20
Systolic Blood Pressure	60-90	70-100	90-110	95-130
Diastolic Blood Pressure	30-55	45-65	50-70	60-80

Purpose

- To assess the patient's condition by comparing temperature, heart rate, respiration and blood pressure readings with the normal standard and previous reading.
- To establish accurate diagnosis, its course and prognosis.
- To prescribe the exact treatment and note its effect.
- Count heart rate, respiration, for one minute each.
- Note temperature in blue dots, heart rate in red dots and respiration with black pencil on the graphic chart.

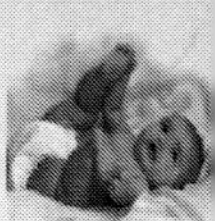

Axillary Temperature

Definition

It means the degree of warmth or balance maintained between the heat produced (Thermogensis) and heat loss (Thermolysis) in the body, compared with a recognized standard. The normal temperature is 37°C or 95°F.

Points to Remember

- Never record oral temperature of infant and children.
- Axilla must be dry for axillary temperature.
- Do not take rectal temperature immediately after administration of enema.
- In order to convert a reading from one scale to the other, the following relationship can be used:

  $(F - 32) \times 5/9 = C$

  $(C \times 9/5) + 32 = F$

Articles Required

Tray Containing

- Thermometer in a container lined with soft material containing disinfectant.
- Container lined with soft material containing plain water.
- Plain swabs in a wide mouthed container.
- Kidney tray and paper bag.

  Graphic (TPR) chart, watch with seconds hand, blue pen.

Steps of the Procedure

1. Explain the procedure to the parents.
2. Take temperature tray to the bedside.
3. Wash your hands.
4. Remove the thermometer from the container containing disfectant and place in the container containing water to rinse.
5. Wipe the thermometer with swab from the bulb to stem in a circular motion and discard the swabs.
6. Read the thermometer and be sure that mercury is below 95°F or 35°C.
7. Dry the axilla.
8. Keep the bulb of the thermometer high in axilla and then hold the young infant's arm against his body for 5 minutes before reading the temperature.
9. Remove and read the thermometer at eye level.
10. Shake down the mercury.

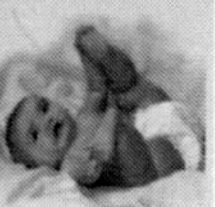

11. Put the thermometer in disinfectant solution and wipe the thermometer from stem to bulb in a circular motion.
12. Then place the thermometer in container with plain water and clean it.
13. Make the patient comfortable.

Rectal Temperature

Tray containing all supplies as for oral temperature, rectal thermometer, instead of oral thermometer little vaseline on a gauze piece.

1. Lubricate the bulb with Vaseline.
2. Turn the patient on your side and place in sim's position.
3. Take two plain swabs in left hand and separate the skin folds around the anus.
4. Introduce the thermometer 4-5 cm with right hand and ask the patient to take a deep breath.
5. Hold the thermometer in place.
6. After one minute remove the thermometer.
7. Wipe it from stem to bulb with swab.
8. Read the thermometer at eye level. Soak the thermometer in disinfectant solution and wipe the thermometer from stem to bulb in a circular motion.

HEART RATE

Definition

The heart rate is a wave of blood created by contraction of the left ventricle of the heart. The rate of pulse is expressed in beats per minute.

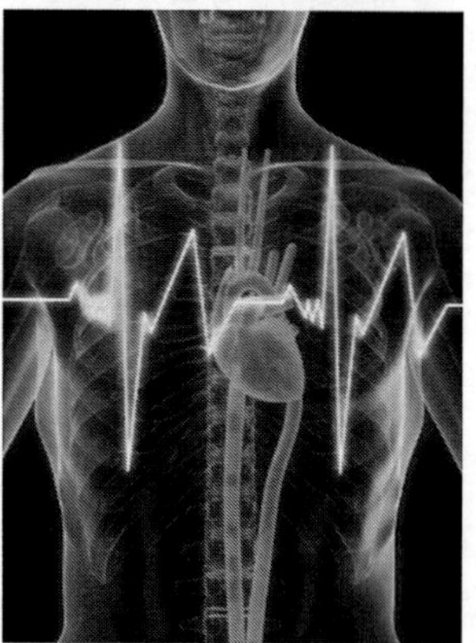

Articles Required

- Watch with second hand, red pen and graphic chart.
- Stethoscope.

Steps of the Procedure

1. Take articles to the bed side.
2. Explain the procedure to the relatives.
3. Wash your hands.
4. Place the patient in supine position or sitting position.
5. Expose the left side of the chest and drape as necessary.
6. Place the stethoscope on the apex of heart midway on the imaginary line drawn from sternum to the left nipple.

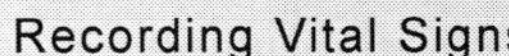

7. Count the heart beats for one full minute.
8. Place the patient in a comfortable position.

RESPIRATION

Definition

It is an involuntary process and consists of inspiration, expiration and pause.

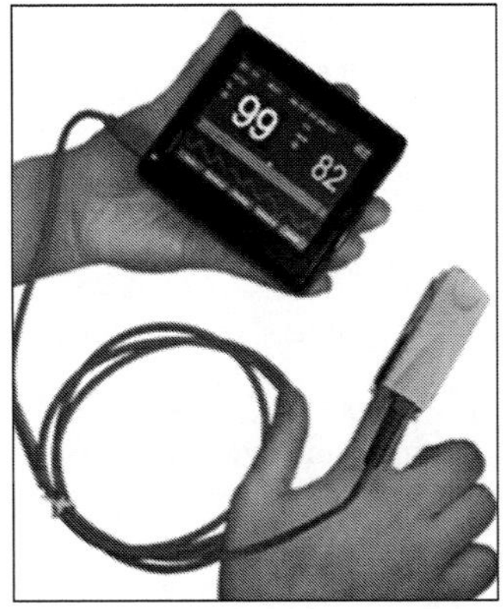

- Infants, 34 to 40 per minute.
- Children aged 1-5 years, 20 to 25 per minute.
- Children older than 5 years, 16 to 20 per minute.

Articles Required

- Watch with second hand, black pencil and graphic chart.

Points to Remember

- Observe the rate and depth of respiration accurately.
- Record immediately after taking heart rate and respiration.

Steps of the Procedure

1. Explain the procedure to the relatives.
2. Make patient comfortable.
3. Count rise and fall of chest or abdomen by watching for full one minute.
4. Record the respiration and mark with black pencil.
5. Report any abnormality.

BLOOD PRESSURE

Definition

It is the lateral pressure exerted by the blood on the walls of blood vessels.

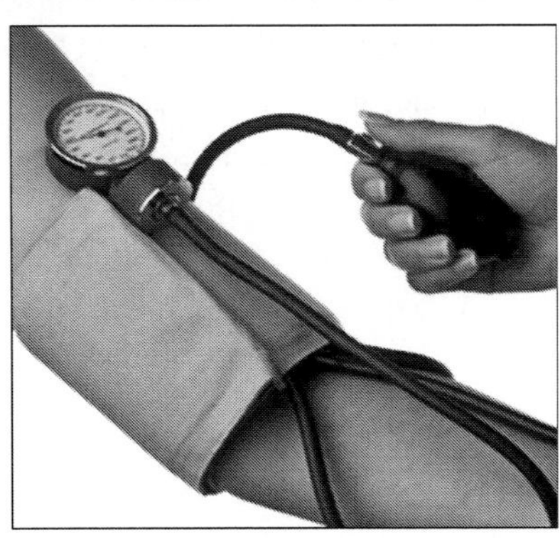

- To measure the blood pressure and to determine the condition of the patient.
- To detect any physiological change in a person.

Points to Remember

- Avoid measuring blood pressure when patient is excited, exhausted or soon after exercise.

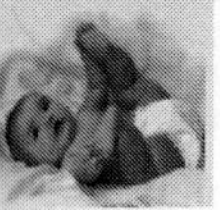

- Keep sphygmomanometer at the level of the patient's heart.
- Make your position to read mercury at eye level.
- Make two readings to make accuracy in measurement.
- Always deflate sphygmomanometer after use.

Articles Required

- Sphygmomanometer.
- Stethoscope.

Steps of the Procedure

1. Explain the procedure to the patient and make him/her comfortable, preferably in lying position.
2. Roll patient's sleeve above elbow.
3. Apply cuff of sphygmomanometer on upper arm smoothly so that lower edge of cuff is 2 cm above antecubital fossa.
4. Keep the arm in a comfortable position.
5. Palpate with fingers the pulsation in the antecubital space.
6. Place stethoscope on the located site.
7. Close the air valve, inflate the cuff until 30 mm of mercury above the point at which you no longer palpate the pulse or it is no longer heard with the stethoscope.
8. Deflate the cuff slowly by opening the air valve gently.
9. Observe the mercury level closely until last sound (softer than before) is heard and record this level of mercury as the diastolic pressure.
10. Release the remaining pressure quickly and repeat procedure for 2nd reading.
11. Report in case of any abnormality.

After Care

- Unwrap the cuff, deflate it.
- Pack the cuff and the pump of the apparatus in a way so that mercury column does not break.
- Replace articles in proper place.
- Record on the patient's chart.

CHAPTER

Collection of Specimen 4

Introduction

Variety of specimen are collected for establishing diagnosis among sick infants. Proper preparation of the patient specimen, collection and handling of the specimen are essential for the production of valid and quality results by a laboratory.

It is essential that the name of the baby/mother's name, date of birth, CR. no and collection time, etc. along with date of collection of specimen must be written.

Definition

Collection of specimens is safe method of obtaining urine, stool, gastric contents and blood for a specific purpose.

Aims of Laboratory Examination

- To make a diagnosis.
- To decide an appropriate course of treatment.
- To assess progress.

General Principles

Before collection of a specimen

- The requested examination and the nature of the specimen should be confirmed from the doctor's laboratory form.
- Proper specimen container should be choosen.
- The label with required particulars should be attached, stating name, CR number, age, unit, ward, name of specimen, the date of collection and time.

Collection of specimen

- Routine specimen should be collected during laboratory working hours, to prevent deterioration.
- For sterile specimens contamination of specimens should be avoided by collecting the specimen straight into a sterile container.

After collecting specimens

- Date and time of collection should be entered on the form.
- The completed label should be attached to the body of the container and upright position should be maintained.

  The written laboratory report should be attached to the record and inform the doctor.

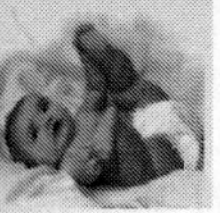

Urine Collection

A Safe method of obtaining urine for a specified purpose.

Purpose

- To check urine for presence of sugar, acetone, bacteria and other urinary products.
- To aid in diagnosis.
- To determine the condition of the patient.
- To determine effectiveness of therapy.

Equipment

Tray with

- Mackintosh with towel.
- Specimen container.
- Wiping agent, e.g. bitadine, normal saline, spirit.
- Gloves: sterile and non sterile.
- Sterile cotton pad.
- Bedpan.
- Kidney tray or paper bag.
- Syringe 5cc with two sterile needle no 24G.

Steps of the Procedure

1. Assess voiding status of client
   - When client last voided.
   - Level of awareness or development stage.
   - Mobility, balance and physical limitations.
2. Assess child's understanding of purpose of test and method of collection.
3. Explain procedure to child or parents.
4. Assemble all the articles at the bed side.
5. Provide the privacy.
6. Perform hand hygiene and wear nonsterile gloves.
7. Position the child so that genitalia are exposed by placing him on his back with legs in frog – like position.
8. Assistance may be needed to hold the legs of the child in proper position.
9. Clean the area in circular motion with betadine then normal saline.
10. If baby is neonate or infant, then attach the urobag in proper position. After voiding, collect the urine in specimen container from bag.

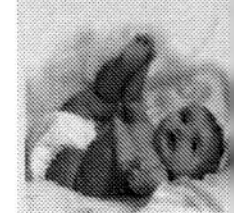

11. Provide the specimen container to parents and explain them to collect urine for routine microscopy when ever the baby voids.
12. Label specimen, write the child's name. CR No. ward, date and time. Attach with laboratory requisition.
13. Write the date, time and put the sign in lab register.
14. Clean the articles and dispose the waste material according to hospital policy.

A midstream urine specimen

The child is explained about the procedure. The child is prepared as above and encouraged to pass the urine into a bed pan. After a small amount has been voided, the midstream urine is directly collected in a sterile wide necked bottle.

Sterile urine specimen

- If the child has a foley's catheter, a sterile specimen can be collected.
- Clamp the catheter near "Y" by artery forceps.
- Wait for 7-8 min.
- Wear the sterile gloves.
- Clean the catheter from above "Y" with betadine and spirit.
- Take the sterile syringe and needle, insert in catheter and aspirate 3-4 ml urine.
- Dispose the old needle and connect the new needle with syringe.
- Collect the urine in sterile container.

Stool Collection

Stool collection is a method of obtaining a stool specimen from the patient.

Purpose

- To check stool for presence of specific material (i.e. blood, Ova, parasites, bacteria or virus)
- To aid in diagnosis.
- To determine condition or status of the patient.
- To determine effectiveness of therapy.

Equipment

- Diaper.
- Plastic liner/mackintosh (used when stool is loose or watery).
- Tongue blade/wooden spatula.
- Specimen container.
- Bedpan.
- Gloves.

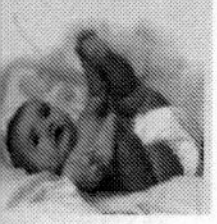

Steps of the Procedure

1. Explain the procedure to the child/parents.
2. Provide privacy.
3. Assemble all the articles at the bed side.
4. If a specimen is needed from a child whose stools are loose or watery enough to be absorbed in the diaper with a piece of plastic. Place thin liner between the diaper and the skin.
5. Wear gloves.
6. Check the child's frequency to see if stooling has occurred.
7. Remove soiled diaper from child. Clean perineal area, apply clean diaper and leave the child comfortable.
8. Remove small amount of stool from diaper with the tongue blade/wooden spatula and place in the specimen container.
9. Label specimen, write the child's name. CR no., ward, date and time. Attach with laboratory requisition.
10. Write the date and time in lab register.
11. Clean the articles and dispose the waste material according to hospital policy.

CHAPTER 5

Restraints

Introduction

Restraints are used to restrict the movements of the sick baby in the bed. The nurse should select appropriate, safe and comfortable restraint. However, the use of restraints should be restricted to the minimum.

Definition

Restraining is the method of immobilizing whole or part of the body of the child to ensure child's safety and/or to facilitate a diagnostic or therapeutic procedure.

Indication

- To ensure a child's safety especially when child has to be left alone.
- To facilitate examination or to carry out procedure safely and effectively.

Restraints can be broadly classified into two-manual and mechanical. Manually restraining the child provides an element of human contact that is lacking in mechanical restraints. When a sedative is administered to facilitate immobilization for a procedure (e.g. infant for an MRI).

Types of Mechanical Restraints

- Mummy restraint.
- Arm and leg restraints.
- Positioning and manual restraining.

Mummy Restraint

When an infant or small child required short-term restraining for examination or treatment that involves the head and neck such as venipuncture, throat examination, gavage feeding, the mummy restraint effectively controls child's movements.

Articles Required

- A blanket or sheet of appropriate size.
- Safety pins or sticking plaster.

Steps of the Procedure

1. Open the blanket or sheet on the bed with one corner folded to the centre.

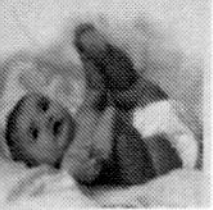

2. Place the infant on the sheet with shoulder at the fold and feet towards the opposite corner.
3. With infant's right arm straight down against the body, the right side of the sheet is pulled across the infant's right shoulder and chest and secured beneath the left side of the body.
4. The left arm is placed straight against the child's side, and the left side of the sheet is brought across the shoulder and chest and locked beneath the child's body on the right side.
5. The lower corner is folded and brought over the body and tucked or fastened securely with safety pins.
6. To modify the mummy restraint for chest examination, the folded edge of the sheet is brought over each arm and under the back, after which the loose edge is folded over and is secured at a point below the chest to allow visualization and access to the chest.

Elbow Restraint

Sometimes it is important to prevent the child from reaching the head or face (e.g. after lip surgery, when a scalp vein infusion is in place, to prevent scratching in skin disorders). For this purpose elbow restraint is used.

A padded cardboard or a spatula is tied along the elbow joint which is placed in anatomical position (arm straight), limiting the movements (flexion) at the joint. Proper length should be selected so that it is long enough to reach comfortably from just below the axilla to the wrist.

Articles Required

A clean tray containing

- Cardboard cut into appropriate size.
- A thin layer of cotton to wrap if spatula is used.
- Bandage to wrap the cardboard or cotton wrapped spatula.
- Sticking plaster to secure the restraint.
- Scissors.
- Paper bag.

Steps of the Procedure

1. Inspect the child and assess the type of restraint required and its size.
2. Assemble the articles and bring them to the bedside.
3. Explain the procedure to child and or to parents. Ensure the need of restraining is understood.
4. Measure the length and cut the cardboard as required.
5. Pad the cardboard with cotton bandage into firm and soft to touch splint.
6. Apply to the joint on the extensor surface.
7. Secure it with the help of a bandage or a plaster.
8. Ensure that the purpose is served.

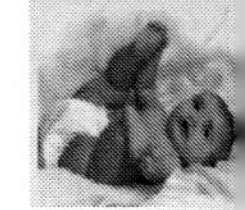

9. Assess the distal pulses and sensation on the extremity.
10. Record and report the procedure.
11. Dissemble the articles.

Points to Remember

- Select the most appropriate restraint according to the age of the child and the purpose of restraining.
- Ensure that the restraint is applied neither too tight nor too loose.
- Frequently assess the restrained extremity for any neurovascular compromise.
- Restraint can be removed for short period of time under constant supervision.
- Repeatedly inform the child (and also ask the parent to tell the child) the rationale behind restraining as he/she may think it as a punishment.
- Inspect the restraint intermittently to ensure that it is serving its purpose.
- Remove restraint as early as possible when the need is over.

CHAPTER 6

Baby Bath

Introduction

Bath time can be an opportunity for the nurse to accomplish much more than general hygiene. It is an excellent time for observation of the infant's behavior such as irritability, State of arousal, alertness and muscular activity. Bathing is done after the vital signs have stabilized. There is no need to immediately wash a newborn, except to remove blood from the face and head.

Definition

Bathing of an infant in a tub/basin.

Purposes

- To wash infant and maintain clean and healthy skin.
- To give infant a chance to exercise and improve circulation.
- To closely observe body for evidence of any abnormalities and to note the infant's growth and development.

Contraindications

- Hypothermia (<36°C).
- Convulsion.
- Bronchopneumonia.
- Congenital cyanotic heart disease.
- Critical illness.
- Premature Infants.

Articles Required

- Vital signs tray.
- A tray containing:
  - Basin-2
  - Soap (Mild)
  - Bath towel
  - Jugs-2
  - Mackintosh

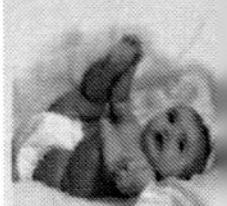

- Face towel
- Sponge clothes (minimum 2)
- Dress
- Bath thermometer
- Swab sticks
- Boiled cooled swabs in a bowl
- Draw sheet
- Kidney tray and paper bag.

- Screen (as per the age of the child).

General Instructions

While giving bath, give mother an opportunity to participate by changing dress, pouring water, etc.

Steps of the Procedure

1. Explain procedure to mother.
2. Assemble necessary articles at bedside.
3. Check infant's temperature.
4. Turn off fan.
5. Check the temperature of water.
6. Place the baby on draw sheet.
7. Pick up 2 boiled cooled swabs, squeeze out the water, simultaneously clean both the eyes. Do not touch the inner surface of the cotton swabs.
8. Dip hand in water and wipe face taking care that no water goes into the infant's mouth.
9. Dry face with face towel. Do not use soap for face.
10. Gently clean the nostrils using swab sticks. Use one swab stick for single nostril.
11. Apply soap gently on the distant arm first, take long strokes.
12. Clean the soap gently on the distant arm first, using the sponge cloth using long strokes.
13. Dry the arm with bath towel.
14. Similarly clean the nearest arm chest and back.
15. Make the baby wear the cloth in the upper half of the body.
16. Change the water if necessary. Maintain the temperature of the water.
17. Now clean the distant leg and the nearest leg.
18. Lastly come to the perineum. Give attention to the groins and the skin folds.
19. Dry the baby nicely and dress him/her.
20. Replace articles.

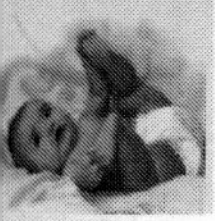

21. Record the time and the condition of the infant.
22. Instruct the mother to feed the infant after bath if not restricted.

NB:

Daily bath may be more harmful than beneficial to the infant by disturbing normal bacterial flora, pH balance, removing essential oils and over drying the skin. Check hospital policy on infant bath.

Ryle's Tube Insertion/Feeding and Removal

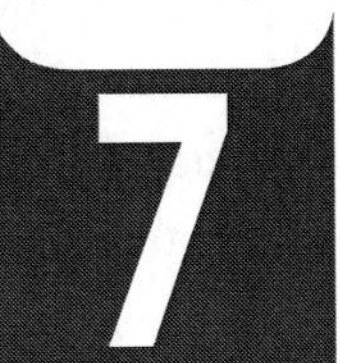

Introduction

When baby is too immature or too sick for well-coordinated sucking, swallowing, esophageal motility and gastric emptying without marked reflux, tube feeding can be used for successful feeding of the baby. Tubes can be passed into the stomach, duodenum or jejunum. Feedings can also be given by continuous infusion.

Definition

This is an alternate method of feeding in which children are fed by a way of tube inserted orally or nasally into the stomach.

Indications

- Diagnostic
  - Evaluation of upper gastrointestinal (GI) bleed (ie, presence, volume).
  - Aspiration of gastric fluid content.
  - Identification of the esophagus and stomach on a chest radiograph.
  - Administration of radiographic contrast to the GI tract.
- Therapeutic
  - Gastric decompression, including maintenance of a decompressed state after endotracheal intubation, often via the oropharynx.
  - Relief of symptoms and bowel rest in the setting of small-bowel obstruction.
  - Aspiration of gastric content from recent ingestion of toxic material.
  - Administration of medication.
  - Feeding.
  - Bowel irrigation.
  - Severe midface trauma.
  - Recent nasal surgery.
  - Relative contraindications.
  - Alkaline ingestion.

Inserting Nasogastric Tube

Articles Required

The articles required for inserting nasogastric tubes are:

- Nasogastric tube: In pediatric patients, the correct tube size varies with the patient's age. To find the correct size, add 16 to the patient's age in years and then divide by 2 (eg, [8 y + 16]/2 = 12F).

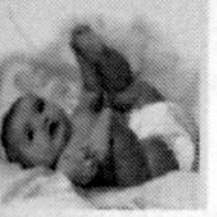

- Mackintosh and draw sheet.
- lidocaine 2% or Saline or warm water to lubricate the tube.
- Stethoscope to check the placement of the tube.
- 5 ml or 10 ml syringe to aspirate the contents.
- A skin friendly tape to secure the tube.
- Kidney Tray.

Steps of the Procedure

1. Explain the procedure, benefits, risks, complications, and alternatives to the patient or the patient's representative.
2. Position the patient as follows:
   - If the patient is awake and alert-in a sitting position in high-Fowler's with the neck partially flexed.
   - If the patient is obtunded or unconscious-head down, preferably in a left side lying position.
   - In new born, the baby can be placed in supine position & nurse can stand on the head end of the babies cot.
3. Place a mackintosh/towel on the patient's chest as well as provide the patient with a basin to minimize contact with aspirated gastric contents.
4. Using the NG tube as a measuring device determine the length of the NG tube to be passed by measuring the length from
   - nose to earlobe
   - earlobe to xiphoid process
   - **NOTE:** in newborn from nose to ear lobe and then earlobe to midpoint of xiphoid process and umbilicus.
5. Add the measurements together and mark this total distance with a small piece of tape.
6. Inspect both of the patient's nostrils for patency.
7. Lubricate the first 6 inches of the NG tube liberally with a water soluble lubricant. Choose the largest patent nostril and begin to pass the NG tube through the nostril to the nasopharynx.
8. Gently insert the nasogastric tube along the floor of the nose and advance it parallel to the nasal floor. Continue to advance the nasogastric tube until the distance of the previously estimated length is reached.
9. No force should be used and if the tube is stuck and resistence is encountered, it should be slightly withdrawn and reinserted.

Verify NG tube placement in the stomach by two of the following:

1. Chest X-ray.
2. Aspirating gastric contents with the irrigation syringe.
3. While listening over the epigastrum with a stethoscope quickly instill a 30cc air bolus with the irrigation syringe. Air entering the stomach will produce a "whooshing" sound.

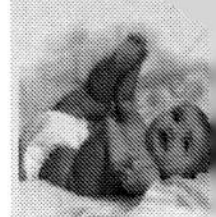

4. Place the open end of the NG tube in a cup of water. Persistent bubbling may indicate that the NG tube has passed through the larynx.
5. If unable to positively confirm that the NG tube has been placed is in the stomach the tube must be removed immediately and re-attempted.
6. Once confirmed for placement, secure the NG tube by placing one end of tape on from the bridge to the tip of the nose and the other end wrapped around the tube itself.

Administering the drug

1. Check prescription for the drug dose, route. Draw the required dose of the liquid drug into an appropriate syringe and place the syringe in a clean receiver.
2. Tablet-crushing must only be considered as a last resort. Check with the pharmacist whether tablets can be crushed, and check your trust's preferred method of tablet-crushing. A tablet-crushing syringe (available from the pharmacy) or pestle and mortar can be used. Crushed tablets can be added to small amount of feed or water and dissolved.
3. Prepare a flush of water in a syringe and label if necessary. Place it in the receiver with the medicines to be administered. Tubes should be flushed before, and after drug administration to prevent interactions between the drugs, tube or feed.
4. Check the patient's identity. Attach the syringe to a port on the enteral feeding tube. Ensure there is an airtight connection between the syringe and enteral tube, and administer the flush and drugs.
5. Flush immediately with an appropriate amount of water and leave the connector clean and dry.

Administering NG feed

1. Collect all the articles near the client bed side.
2. Confirm with the client's file the amount & type of feed to be given.
3. Confirm that the feed should not be hot.
4. Raise the head end of the bed.
5. Wash hands.
6. Explain the procedure to the client or parents.
7. Check bowel sounds & confirm the placement of the tube in the stomach.
8. Spread draw sheet on the chest of the client.
9. Wear clean gloves.
10. Attach syringe to the NG tube of the client & flush it with 10ml of water.
11. Pour measured amount of feed into NG tube & let it flow by gravity.
12. Observe the clients activity to be sure he/she is comfortable if not then stop the procedure.
13. Flush the tube after the feed with 10ml of water.
14. Put cap on the end of the tube to make it air tight again.
15. Chart the type, amount, quantity of feed given & replace the articles.

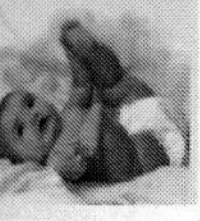

After Care

A. Patient

- Before leaving ensure that patient is in comfortable position.

B. Articles

- Terminate the procedure properly.
- Replace the articles after washing.

REMOVING NASOGASTRIC TUBE

Points to Remember

- Confirm the physician order to remove the tube.
- Assess for the presence of bowel sounds.
- Assess for the absence of nausea or vomiting when tube is clamped.

Articles Required

The articles required for removing nasogastric tube are:

- A clean tray containing.
- Clean gloves.
- 5 ml syringe.
- Gauze pieces.
- Mackintosh and small towel/draw sheet.
- Screen.
- Plastic disposable bag.

Steps of the Procedure

1. Explain to the patient what you are going to do, why it is necessary and how he or she can cooperate. Explain that the procedure will cause no discomfort.
2. Assist the patient to a sitting position if health permits.
3. Place mackintosh and draw sheet across the patient chest to collect any spillage of mucous and gastric secretions from the tube.
4. Wash hands and put on clean gloves.
5. Provide privacy.
6. Remove the adhesive tape securing the tube to the nose.
7. Instill 5 ml of air into the tube to clear the tube of any contents such as feeding or gastric drainage.
8. Ask the patient to take deep breath and hold it. This will close the glottis thereby preventing accidental aspiration of any gastric contents.

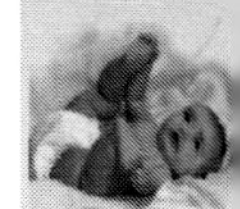

9. Pinch the tube with the gloved hands. This will prevent any content inside the tube from draining into the patient's throat.
10. Quickly and smoothly withdraw the tube.
11. Place the tube in the plastic bag and observe the intactness of the tube.
12. Provide mouth care if the patient desires and help him to clean the nasal secretions.

After Care:

- Terminate the procedure properly.
- Replace the articles after washing.

CHAPTER 8

Spoon and Katori Feeding

Introduction

When the spoon is first introduced to infants they are likely to push it away and appear dissatisfied. Some patience and skill is required to overcome this initial response, especially if the extrusion reflex is still present.

The spoon feeding should be attempted before and after ingestion of a small amount of breast milk or formula to associate this new experience with a pleasurable and satisfying experience.

Each new food is introduced at intervals of 4 to 7 days to allow identification of food allergies.

"Feeding with a spoon and katori has been found to be safe in low birth weight babies this mode of feeding is a bridge between gavage feeding and direct breast feeding".

Definition

This is the method used for feeding when the infant cannot latch on to the mother because either the mother or the infant is sick.

Articles Required

- Face towel.
- Katori, spoon.
- Feed of required amount.
- Mackintosh and towel.

Steps of the Procedure

1. Assemble the required articles at bedside.
2. Explain the procedure to the mother (if present).
3. Wash hands.
4. Hold the child in your lap to achieve better control, (the child can be restrained in a blanket or sit with his right arm under your (Nurse's) left arm.
5. Check the temperature of the feed by dropping 1-2 drops on the back of the hand before taking the child in your lap.
6. Place mackintosh and towel below the chin of the child.
7. Hold the katori and pour few drops of feed by spoon on the tongue of the baby to stimulate secretion of digestive juice and then give required amount of feed.

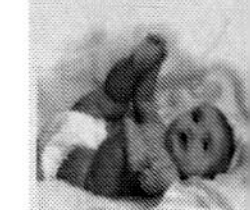

8. Continue giving spoon filled, with optimum interval between each feed. Give time to the child in between the feed to rest if the child is crying. Burp in between as and when needed.
9. Clean the mouth after the feed finishes.
10. Record the feedings with time amount and date.

After Care

- Clean, dry and replace them for reuse.

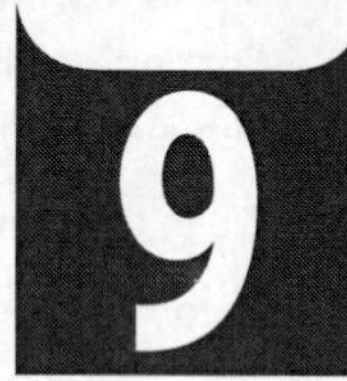

Gastrostomy/Jejunostomy Feeding

Introduction

Gastrostomy is a widely used route of feeding when long term nutrition is indicated. Children having congenital abnormalities such as Tracheoesophsgeal fistula, atresia and children with esophageal injuries (e.g. ingestion of caustic chemicals).

Direct operative access to the small bowel for feeding purposes is almost as old as that approach to the stomach. However, Jejunostomies are not used as frequently as Gastrostomies because they are more difficult to place and maintain.

Jejunostomy can be divided into short, medium and long-term access, regarding their expected length of use. These can also be divided into indirect and direct jejunal access depending upon how the catheter is placed.

Definition

Gastrostomy/Jejunostomy feeding is a method of maintaining hydration and nutrition for patients, who are not able to take in an adequate oral intake to maintain nutritional status. A feeding tube is passed directly into the patient's stomach through the abdominal wall (gastrostomy) or into the small intestine (Jejunostomy) to administer fluid feed.

Gastrostomy tubes are usually 12-30 G and have a balloon, mushroom tip or disk securing internally. Externally the tube has a disk or bumper at skin level and at the distal end an adapter that connects to a feeding tube or syringe and has a side port for medication administration. Jejunostomy tubes are placed through the abdominal wall into the jejunum either directly or via the stomach (gastro jejunostomy). They are used when the patient has a high-risk of aspiration. Jejunostomy tubes are usually 8-24 G.

Indication

- Children in whom passage of tube through mouth, pharynx, esophagus, and cardiac sphincter is contraindicated or impossible.
- Intact GIT but unable to consume sufficient calories to meet nutritional needs.
- Impaired swallowing related to neurological conditions, obstruction related to neoplasm or surgery.
- Surgery of upper GIT.
- Children require tube feeding for an extended period of time (to avoid the constant irritation by an NG tube).

Articles Required

- A clean tray containing.
- 50 ml syringe to aspirate gastric contents.
- Enteral feeding bag with tubing if administering bag feed.

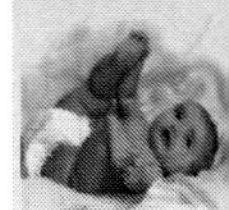

- I/V set with burette if administering a continuous feed.
- Enteral pump and compatible line if administering feed via a pump.
- 50 ml syringe if administering bolus feed via syringe.
- Water for flushing.
- Warm prepared formula feed.
- Measuring cup to measure the feed.
- Medications, powdered if to be given.
- Mackintosh with towel to avoid soiling of bed and clothes of the patient.
- Gauze pieces in a bowl to clean the skin if wet.
- Kidney tray and paper bag to discard the waste.

Steps of the Procedure

1. Verify the feeding instruction by the physician.
2. Assemble the articles and bring them to the bedside.
3. Explain the procedure to the child and/or to the parent/ relative.
4. Give the child semi-Fowler position.
5. Wash hands and dry them.
6. Spread the mackintosh with towel.
7. Aspirate the tube and see for the residual volume.
8. Measure and take the required quantity of warm feed.
9. Pour warm feed into 50 ml feeding syringe hold it high allowing it to flow slowly by gravity. Or use a drip set and hang the bottle containing required amount of feed; as per physician's instruction.
10. To administer as bolus, attach the syringe to the gastrostomy/jejunostomy tube and inject slowly.
11. If a mechanical pump is used, set the pump flow rate after attaching the syringe containing the required quantity of feed so that the feed is administered at a slow and steady rate.
12. Flush the tube with 2-5-10 ml of water (according to the age of the child) to clear the tube off feed.
13. Clamp the tube.
14. Clean the skin if wet.
15. Remove the mackintosh and towel.
16. Comfort the child in semi-fowler or on right side for at least 1 hour.
17. Record the feeding including characteristic of residual aspirated, quantity and type of formula given along with the time and signature of the person who administered feed.
18. Dissemble the articles.

Points to Remember

- Aspirate the residual gastric content before the next feed. If the quantity is more than half of the previous feed notify the physician. Otherwise push it back and subtract from the quantity of feed to be administered if significant.
- Warm the feed to room temperature before administering.
- Maintain fowlers/semi-fowler position while feeding and for at least for one hour.

CHAPTER 10

Oral Medication

Introduction

The oral route is preferred for administering/medications to children whenever possible. Because of the ease of administration of oral medications. It must be dissolved or suspended in liquid preparations. Although, some children are able to swallow or chew solid medication at an early age, solid preparations are not recommended for young children because of the danger of aspiration.

Definition

It is the process of administering prescribed medications orally.

Purpose

To provide a medication that has systemic effect on gastrointestinal tract.

Articles Required

- Tablets, powders with respective container and proper label.
- Syrups in bottle with tight cover.
- Mortar and pestle.
- Measuring cup/glass/katori.
- Treatment chart.
- Small mackintosh with towel.
- Small plastic cups or paper bags.
- Spoon.
- Water.
- Kidney tray/paper bag.

Steps of the Procedure

1. Explain the procedure to child/parents.
2. Determine Physician's orders and patient.
3. Assess the medical history, allergy history, diet history.
4. Gather physical examination and laboratory data.
5. Assemble all the articles in tray near bedside.

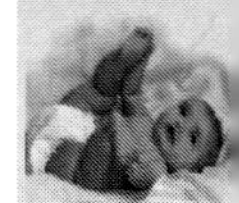
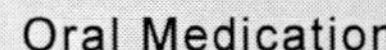

6. Check the Ten Rights of medication administration
   - Right Patient Regarding to the right patient to be administered a medication.
   - Right Medication Regarding to the right medication to be administered to a patient.
   - Right Dosage Right and enough dose.
   - Right Route Medication should take on it's real time matter of way. (if must to be taken oral, it should be taken orally.)
   - Right Time Should be according on right time.
   - Right Documentation Right input of information, data, and details.
   - Right Client Education Right health teaching.
   - Right to Refuse Right to reject medication.
   - Right Assessment Right to determine real illness. (examination)
   - Right Evaluation Right examination and right judgment. (finalized examination)

1. Calculate correct dose. Take time and double check calculations.
2. Check the expiry date of medicine.
3. Place all medicines in one cup, if child has difficulty in swallowing, crush tablets in mortal and pestle (Do not crush enteric coated tablets)
4. For preparing liquids, shake bottle and hold medication cup to eye level and pour medicine to desired level in measuring cup.
5. Assist child to comfortable position.
6. Spread towel/draw sheet under the chin.
7. Place medication in mouth against cheeks and provide water to swallow or give dissolved medicines or liquid medicines to swallow.
8. Give child a flavoured ice pops or small candy in between administration of different drugs.
9. For medications with unpleasant taste or smell, have child pinch the nose and drink the medicine through a straw.
10. Infants should be given medications in needle less syringe or dropper 0.25 ml – 0.50 ml at a time.
11. Clean, dry and replace the articles.
12. Record the medication administration with date, time and signature.

Points to Remember

- Do not give water after administering cough syrups.
- While pouring the liquid medicine, do not pour it from the label side.
- For giving medicine, hold the child in semi reclining position to prevent aspiration.
- Child may be allowed to suck medication through disposable syringe or nipple.
- Once medication is emptied in patient's mouth, blow a small puff of air on to the face to elicit swallowing reflex.

Intravenous Infusion

Introduction

An intravenous infusion (I/V) is the instillation of large amount of fluids, electrolytes, or nutrient substances into a vein. It is given to patients who require extra fluid or those who cannot take fluids or nutrient substances orally Venous access allows the sampling of blood, as well as administration of fluids, medications, parenteral nutrition, chemotherapy, and blood products Pediatric intravenous infusion is an integral part of modern medicine and is practiced in virtually every health care setting.It is the responsibility of the nurse to carry out the physician's order by correctly and effectively starting the I/V infusion and by regulating the desired flow rate.

Definition

The introduction of a large amount of fluid into the body via veins is termed as intravenous infusion.

Purpose

- To restore the fluid volume that is lost from the body due to hemorrhage, vomiting, diarrhea, drainage, etc.
- To meet the patient's basic requirements for calories, water, minerals and vitamins.
- To prevent and treat shock and collapse.
- To supply the body with nourishment and fluid when oral intake is contraindicated.
- To supply whole blood, or more of blood's components.
- To administer drugs in large volume preparation (e.g. Metrogyl, Vancomycin)

Types of Fluids used for Intravenous Infusion

- For initial 2 days 10% dextrose is administered.
- Na & K are added later on on 3rd day and 4th day of life.
- KCl is added (2mmol/kg/day) to maintenance IV fluid from 3rd day of life.

Other Fluids used are

- Dextrose 5%, 20% etc.
- Normal Saline 0.9%, 0.45%.
- Isolyte P.
- DNS.
- Amino acids.

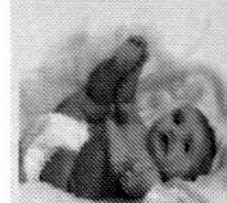

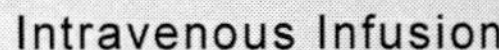

- Vitamins, lipids.
- Blood plasma.
- Drugs: for example, Mannitol, Metrogyl, etc.

Articles Required

- I/V stand.

A tray containing

- I/V solutions.
- Sterile I/V tubing with drip chamber and clamp.
- Sterile butterfly or scalp vein needle /IV cannula (vein flown) of appropriate size.
- Sterile syringes (To take blood specimen).
- Sterile cotton swabs in a sterile covered container.
- Sterile dissecting forceps in a sterile bottle.
- Gauze pieces.
- Spirit.
- Mackintosh with cover.
- Tourniquet.
- Kidney tray and paper bag.
- Adhesive plaster and scissors.
- Splint.

Steps of the Procedure

1. Explain the procedure to the child or parents, restrain children, select a site (basalic and cephalic veins, saphenous).
2. Wash hands, remove the bottle seal from the top, clean the top with spirit swab, holding the bottle upright, insert the drip set and air went into the bottle.
3. Close the clamp and hang the bottle on the I/V stand about 18-25" high.
4. Connect the needle to the I/V tubing. Open the clamp and flush the I/V fluid through the tubing and needle into the kidney tray until air is removed. Clamp the tubing again, apply protective cap over the needle.
5. Prepare few strips of adhesive tapes.
6. Site preparation: apply tourniquets firmly 6 to 8"proximal to the site.
7. Stabilize the vein using your nondominant hand (thumb) applying traction to the skin distal to the chosen site of insertion. This will prevent superficial veins from rolling away from the needle. Stabilization should be maintained throughout the procedure.
8. Clean the area with a spirit swab.

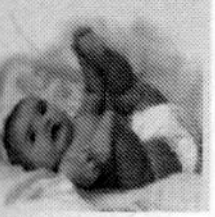

9. Insert the I/V cannula into the vein at 15-30o angle and once it enters the vein, make it parallel with the skin and follow the course of the vein.
10. When back flow of blood occurs into the needle and its hub, insert the needle further into the vein about ¾ to 1".
11. Cap the I/V access to prevent blood loss.
12. Release the tourniquet.
13. Secure the I/V cannula with adhesive strips.
14. Immobilize with splint.
15. Connect the I/V line to the I/V access (cannula/scalp vein).
16. Open the clamp to let the fluid run.
17. Set the flow rate and recheck it, once or twice.
18. Record in nurses' notes and intake – output chart.
19. Dissemble the articles.

General Instruction

- Maintain strict aseptic technique.
- Be sure of solutions types.
- Avoid entry of air.
- Clamp, before the whole amount of fluid finishes.
- Check the apparatus for the working condition
- Observe the site for swelling (tissue infiltration), leaking and bleeding.
- Observe the patient for unfavorable symptoms.
- Regulate the flow of fluid.

Holiday Segar Formula for Calculation of fluid requirement

Weight	Baseline Daily Fluid Requirement
10 Kg	100 ml/kg body weight
11-20 Kg	1000 + 50 ml/kg for each kg over 10 kg
Over 20 Kg	1500 ml + 20 ml/kg for each kg over 20 kg

For Example for 13 Kg

= 1000 ml + 3 x 50 ml

=1150 ml

Fluids to be increased in presence of

- Increased weight loss.
- Decreased urine output.
- Increased serum sodium.

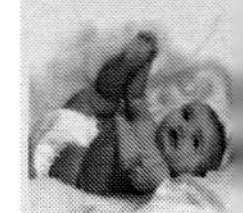

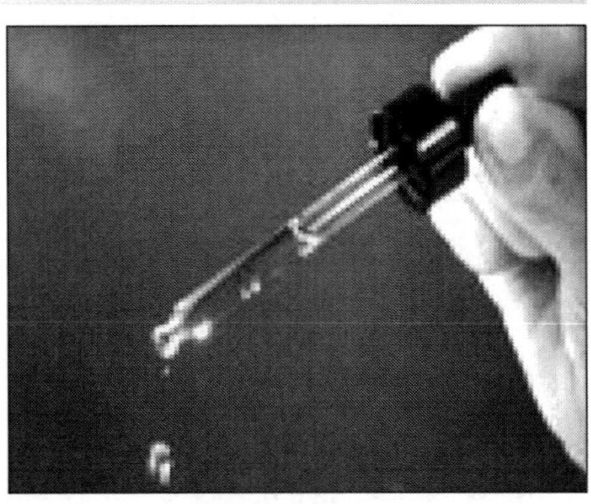

- Increased urine specific gravity.
- Radiant warmer or Phototherapy.

Fluids to be increased in presence of

- Excessive Weight gain.
- Renal Failure.
- Decreased serum sodium.
- Decreased urine specific gravity

For Example, $\frac{300(\text{ml}) \times 16}{4 \times 60}$ = 20 drops/min

(4 hr = 4×60 min)

Example: Calculate the hourly maintenance fluid rate for a child who weighs 25 kg

(100 mL x 10 kg) + (50 mL x 10 kg) + (20 mL x 5 kg)/24 hrs

(1000 mL) + (500 mL) + (100 mL) = 1600 mL/24 hrs = 66.7 ml/hr

Using this formula the hourly fluid maintenance for this child is 67 mL/hr

– Flow rate depends on condition and need of the child, his/her weight and nature of the fluid. Warm the fluid to room temperature before administering.

IV Catheter Removal

1. Stop the infusion and disconnect tubing leaving just the saline/heparin lock tubing connected to the venous access device.
2. Release the adhesive tape and transparent dressing from the skin.
3. Withdraw the catheter outside of the vein and apply direct pressure with gauze for at least 5 minutes.
4. Inspect the catheter for fragmentation and document in the patient's chart the date, time, and reason for catheter removal and the integrity of the catheter as inspected.
5. Place a 2 × 2 gauze pad or a cotton ball with a paper tape over the intravenous insertion site and instruct the patient to continue manual pressure for 10 more minutes in order to minimize hematoma formation.

CHAPTER 12

Intravenous Injection

Introduction

Intravenous is a term that means within the vein. Thus, is the introduction of a medication into the veins necessary for treatment purpose.

Definition

Medicines and fluids when introduced into a vein using needle is called Intravenous Injection.

Purpose

- To get rapid and systemic effect of the drug.
- To provide the needed effect even when the patient is unconscious.
- Assures that the total dosage will be administered and the same will be absorbed for the systemic action of the drug.
- Provides only means of administration for medications that cannot be given orally.

General Instruction

- Give injections only on the doctor's written orders.
- Follow strict aseptic techniques.
- Observe the "seven rights" of the administrations of medicine.
- Never use a drug whose expiry date is over.
- Always have the patient relaxed and placed in a comfortable position.
- Expel the air from the syringe before the injection.

Nurse's Responsibility in the Administration of Intravenous Injection

Preliminary Assessment

- Check the diagnosis and age of the patient.
- Check the purpose of injection.
- Check the physician's order.
- Check the patient's name, bed number and other identification.

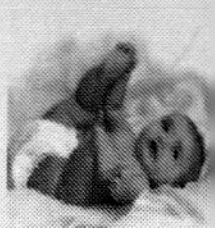

Articles Required

A tray containing

- Syringes and needles
- Sterile gauze piece
- Spirit swabs
- Kidney tray
- Distilled water
- Drug ordered
- Filer

Preparation of Patient and Environment

- Identify the patient correctly.
- Explain the procedure to the patient.
- Restraint the site of injection.
- As far as possible avoid meal timings.
- Keep attention of the patient away from the injection by friendly conversations.

Steps of the Procedure

1. Select the medication
2. Wash hands.
3. Prepare the medication
4. Select the appropriate syringe.
5. Select the solvent.
6. Recheck the order, treatment chart with the label of medicine, expiry date, etc.
7. Calculate the dosage of the medication, the amount of solvent to be added to obtain the required dosage.

$$\text{Drug to administerted} = \frac{\text{Require Dose (mg)} \times \text{Amount of solvent (ml)}}{\text{Total Dose (mg)}}$$

   - Take the solvent in the syringe and introduce it into the vial.
   - Mix the powder with the solvent by rotating the vial in the palm of hand.
   - When mixed well, take out the required amount of solution in the syringe.

Prepare the Site for Injection

- Clean the cannula with spirit swab.
- Place sterile gauze piece under the cannula.
- Flush the cannula with distilled water.

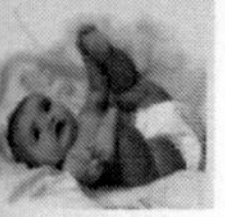

- Inject the drug slowly.
- Flush the cannula with distilled water.

Dosage Calculation

Young's formula

$$\frac{\text{Age of the child in year} \times \text{Adult does}}{\text{Age of the child in year} + 12}$$

Clark's formula

$$\frac{\text{Weight of the child pounds} \times \text{Adult dose}}{150}$$

After Care of the Patient and Articles

- Help the patient to dress up and take a comfortable position.
- Watch for the signs and symptoms of allergic reaction.
- Take all articles in duty room. Wash with cold water first and then with warm soapy water.
- Clean all other articles and replace them in their proper places.
- Wash hands.
- Record the procedure on the nurse's record.

Intramuscular Injection

Introduction

Injections of any kind can hurt; children know that pain is predictable. Preparation for an intramuscular injection should be done just before giving the injection, so that children do not have time to build up their anxieties about the procedure. The pediatric nurse needs to be competent enough to give intramuscular injections.

Definition

Medication when injected into the muscles, is called intramuscular injection.

Purposes of Injection

- To get a rapid and systemic effect of the drug.
- To help in quick absorption than oral drug.
- To provide means of administration for medication that cannot be given orally or I/V
- To provide the needed effect even when the child is unconscious/very small or unable to swallow/ when peripheral line is not accessible.

Different Sites of giving Intramuscular Injections

- **Vastus lateralis:** Palpate to find greater trochanter and knee joints, divide vertical distance between these two landmarks into three equal parts, inject into middle one-third.
- **Ventrogluteal:** Palpate to locate greater trochanter, anterior superior iliac tubercle and posterior iliac crest: place palm of hand over greater trochanter, index finger over anterior superior iliac tubercle and middle finger along crest of ilium, posteriorly as far as possible inject into centre of "V" formed by fingers.
- **Dorsogluteal:** Locate greater trochanter and postetior superior iliac spine, draw imaginary line between these two points and inject into lateral and superior to line into gluteus maximus or medius muscle.
- **Deltoid:** Locate acromian process, inject only into upper third of muscle that begins about two finger breadths below acromian but is above axilla.

Determining the Site

Factors that are considered when selecting site for an IM injection on an infant or child include the following:

- The amount and character of the medicine to be injected.
- The amount and general condition of the muscle mass.

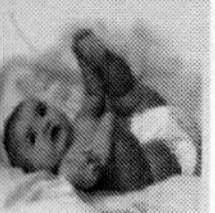

- The frequency or number of injection to be given during the course of treatment.
- Factors that may impede across or cause contamination of the site.
- The child's ability to assume the required position safely.

Articles Required

- Sterile tray with sterile gauze piece lining for injection.
- Syringe and appropriate size needle (23/24 G).
- Extra needle (20/22 G), if medication is drawn from vial.
- Spirit swabs.
- Injection in the form of vial or ampule.
- Ampule cutter.
- Medication card.
- Kidney tray and paper bag.

Steps of the Procedure

1. Arrange all articles at the bed side.
2. Check medicine card with patient's chart for name, hospital number, drug to be administered, dosage, route of administration and time of administration (7R).
3. Prepare medication from ampule or vial asceptically. Be sure that all air is expelled.
4. Provide privacy (if the child is older).
5. Explain to mother/child.
6. Assess the site of giving IM injection.
7. Position and expose appropriate site.
8. Locate the anatomical site for giving IM injection.
9. Clean the site with cotton swab moistened with spirit.
10. Ensure that the site is dry.
11. Grasp the body of muscle between thumb and fingers.
12. Secure and hold the child firmly.
13. Insert the needle quickly at 90° into muscles.
14. Withdraw the piston and push the injection slowly.
15. Talk to the child during the procedure.
16. Quickly remove the needle and apply firm pressure. Do not massage.
17. Give the child comfortable position.
18. Discard the waste properly as per the biomedical waste disposal rules.
19. Observe the site for any bleeding, redness.

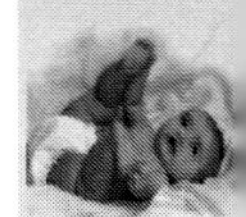

20. Record date, time and name of the drug, dosage and route in nurse's record. Full signature of nurse is mandatory.

Complications of Injection

- Induration.
- Allergic reactions.
- Infection.
- Pyogenic reaction.
- Pain.
- Trauma.
- Psychological stress.
- Over dosage or under dosage.
- Errors in the administration of medication.

Note: Do not recap the used disposable needle.

Do not bend, break, or otherwise manipulate used needles by hand.

CHAPTER

Steam Inhalation

Introduction

As children and infants are very small and they do not follow instructions, it is important for the nurse to be very conscious while giving steam inhalation.

Definition

It is the process in which water is boiled to steam which is inhaled through nose and mouth for therapeutic purpose.

Purposes

- To relieve congestion and inflammation.
- To loosen the thick secretion.
- To decrease edema of the respiratory tract.
- To help in expectoration.
- To aid in absorption of oxygen.
- To relieve spastic condition of larynx and bronchi.
- To provide heat and moisture and to prevent dryness of mucus membrane.

Articles Required

A Tray Containing

- Swab sticks.
- Face towel.
- Kettle containing boiled water.
- Blanket.
- Sputum mug with antiseptic lotion.

Preliminary Preparation

- Make sure that the child has not taken cold drinks just before giving steam.
- Switch off the fans to prevent draught.
- Fill the kettle half and plug the cable to the electric connection, boil the water till the steam is produced.
- Never keep the kettle on the bed. Always keep it on the chair.

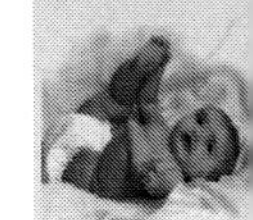

- As per the child's age give him instruction so that he could follow.
- If the infant is your client and he starts crying automatically, the child will inhale steam.
- Never leave the child alone. Let the parents be with the child while taking steam.

Steps of the Procedure

1. Arrange all articles at the bed side.
2. Wash hands.
3. Switch off the fan.
4. Clean the nostrils of the child.
5. Make the child sit on his parent's lap at one edge of the bed.
6. Put the kettle on the chair at one side of the bed.
7. Cover the child with bed sheet and tell him to take the steam.
8. Give him steam for approximately 10-15 minutes till the steam is coming. Make sure that the water is boiled enough to produce steam.
9. Give chest physiotherapy.
10. Instruct the child to cough if he can follow the instructions.
11. Wipe off the steam on his face.
12. Dismantle all articles and wash hands.
13. Do recordings in the nurse's notes.

CHAPTER 15

Endotracheal Suctioning

Introduction

Suctioning is the aspiration of secretions, through suction catheter connected to a suction machine. It is recommended that sterile techniques be used for all suctioning, so that microorganisms are not introduced into the pharynx, where they can multiply and move into trachea and bronchi. The suction apparatus includes a collection bottle, a tubing system connected to suction catheter, and a gauge that registers the degree of suction. Oropharyngeal or nasopharyngeal suctioning removes secretions from the upper respiratory tract. Deeper suctioning called Endotracheal Suctioning, removes secretions from trachea and the bronchi.

Definition

Endotracheal suctioning is a procedure done to remove secretion from trachea and bronchi and facilitate respiration.

Purposes

- To remove secretions that obstructs the airway.
- To facilitate respiratory ventilation.
- To obtain secretions for diagnostic purposes.
- To prevent infection that may result from accumulated secretions.

Indications

If Child is

- Unable to expectorate coughed secretions.
- Unable to swallow.
- Makes light bubbling or rattling breath sounds.
- Restlessness.
- Adventitious breath sound when chest is auscultated.
- Change in mental status, skin color, rate and pattern of respirations, pulse and rhythm.

General Instruction

- Gentle suctioning is necessary to prevent laryngospasm, reflex bradycardia, and other cardiac arrhythmias from vagal stimulation.

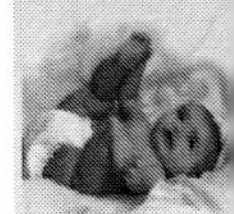

- If nasal suctioning is necessary it must be done after oral suctioning to minimize possibility of aspiration of oropharyngeal content.
- Proper vacuum pressure and suction catheter size are important to prevent atelectasis and decrease hypoxia from suctioning procedure.
- Vacuum pressure should range from 60 to 100 mm Hg for infants and children and from 40 to 60 mm Hg for preterm infants.
- Unless secretions are thick and tenacious, the lower range of negative pressure is recommended.
- Suctioning should not be performed for more than 5 seconds duration.
- Counting one-one thousand, two-one thousand, three-one thousand, and so on while suctioning is a simple means for monitoring the time. Hyper oxygenating, hyperventilating the child with 100% oxygen before and after suctioning must be ensured.

Preliminary Assessment

- Check the diagnosis and age of patient.
- Check the purpose of suction.
- Check the physician's orders for type of suctioning, time and route of suctioning.
- Check the patient's name, bed no. and other identification.
- Check the nurse's record to find the time at which the last suction was done.
- Check the necessity for suctioning.

Articles Required

A tray containing

- Sterile suction catheter.
- 8-10 Fr for children.
- 5-8 Fr for infants.
- Sterile gloves.
- Normal saline bottle.
- Sterile gauze.
- Portable or wall suction machine with tubing.
- Sputum trap.
- Kidney tray.

Preparation of Patient and Environment

- Identify the patient correctly.
- Explain procedure to the patient's attendant.
- Restrain the baby/child physically.
- Suctioning should be done before feeding.
- Give proper position to patient.

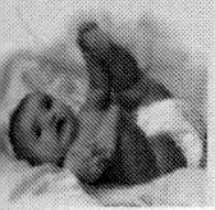

- Take all articles to bedside.
- Check suction apparatus is in working condition and attach suction catheter with sterile wrapper to suction tubing.
- Preoxygenation before suctioning should be done.

Steps of the Procedure

1. Wash hands.
2. Put on sterile gloves.
3. Maintain sterility of dominant gloved hand.
4. With sterile gloved hand pick up the catheter.
5. Test the pressure of suction and patency of catheter by applying your sterile gloved finger.
6. Detach the oxygen tubing from ET tube with nondominant hand.
7. With dominant hand insert the suction catheter into ET tube gently till resistance is felt.
8. While inserting the catheter place thumb at opening.
9. After insertion release thumb and suction for 5 seconds and rotate the catheter gently.
10. Take out the catheter while rotating gently.
11. Attach oxygen tubing and do chest physiotherapy.
12. SpO_2 is increased by 10 - 20% above baseline during suctioning.
13. Monitor SpO_2 pulse and respiration.
14. Allow 20-30 seconds intervals between each suction.
15. Wipe off the catheter with sterile gauze.
16. Flush the catheter with sterile water.
17. Repeat the procedure until the secretions are minimal.

After care of Patient and Articles

- Assist the client to a comfortable position.
- Dispose of catheter, gloves and gauze pieces.
- Auscultate the client's breathing sounds to ensure they are clear of secretions.
- Observe skin color, dyspnea and level of anxiety.
- Document the time, amount, color, consistency and odor of sputum.

CHAPTER 16

Oxygen Therapy

Oxygen Therapy

Supplemental oxygen is used to treat medical conditions in which the tissues of body do not have enough oxygen. Oxygen therapy is the administration of oxygen as a medical intervention, which can be for a variety of purposes in both chronic and acute patient care. It is one of the most common procedures carried out in the management of children with respiratory diseases & other illnesses.

Indications

1. **Hypoxic Hypoxia:** The basic defect is that less O_2 reaches blood. It may be due to Low O_2 conc. in air e.g. high altitudes.
2. **Anemic Hypoxia:** When capacity of blood to carry O_2 is reduced. It may be due to Low Hb content in blood.
3. **Demand Hypoxia:** When O_2 utilization by tissues is faster & more than supply of O_2. It occurs during Hyperpyrexia.
4. **Ischemic Hypoxia:** When blood reaching tissues is less or slower than normal blood supply. It can occur due to low cardiac output.

Histotoxic hypoxia: The fault is at cellular level so the tissues are not able to utilize O_2 available to them e.g. Septicemia, Poisoning.

Oxygen delivery Equipments: All systems require.

1. Oxygen supply.
2. Flow meter.
3. Oxygen tubing.
4. Delivery device.
5. Humidifier.

Methods of O_2 therapy

1. Non invasive.
2. Invasive.

Non invasive devices

1. Nasal cannula.
2. Face mask.

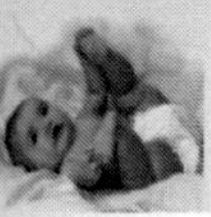

3. O_2 tent.
4. Mask with reservoir bag.
5. Venturi mask.
6. O_2 hood.

Invasive devices

1. Nasal catheter.
2. ET tube.
3. Tracheotomy tube.

Low flow system: It cannot meet the total inspiratory requirement of the patient.

High flow system: It can provide the flow rate sufficient to meet patient requirement needed for assisted or controlled ventilation.

O_2 therapy devices: Non invasive devices

1. **Nasal cannula**

   The nasal cannula (NC) is a thin tube with two small prongs that are inserted inside anterior nares that protrude into the patients nostrils.

   - Cause less irritation to patient.
   - 1 to 6 L/min of oxygen fio$_2$ 25 to 50%.

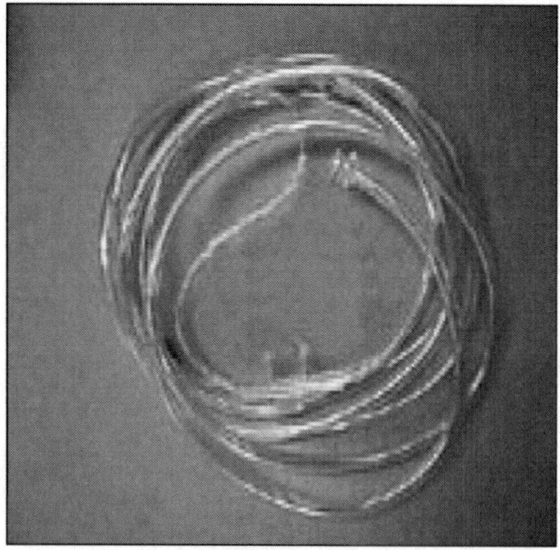

Nasal cannula

2. **Face mask**
   - Available in various sizes and types.
   - Can be held in place by rubber head band.
   - Mask of proper size should be used.

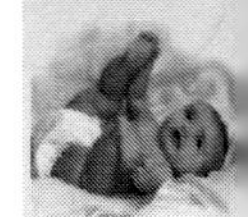

- Mask with 6 to 12 L/min of O_2 fio_2 is 35 to 55% but if attached with reservoir bag fio_2 is up to 95 to 100%.
- The final oxygen concentration delivered by this device is dependent upon the amount of room air that mixes with the oxygen the patient breathes.
- Well tolerated by patients.

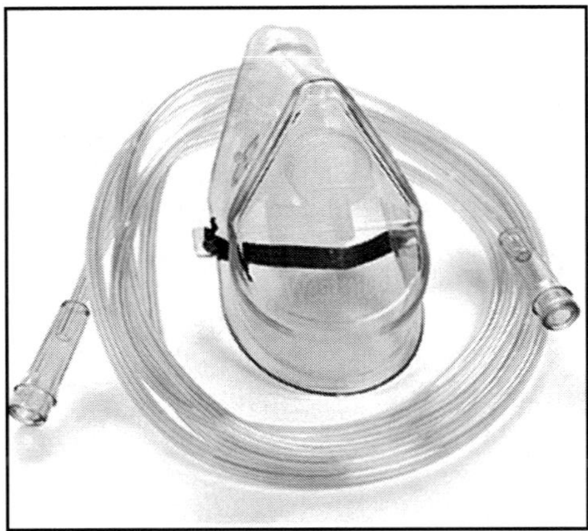

Face Mask

4. **Partial Rebreathing Mask:**
   - Mask with reservoir.
   - Delivers 35-60% Oxygen at 6-10 L/min flow rate.
   - First third of exhaled gases mix with reservoir.
   - Exhaled gases from upper airway are oxygen rich.

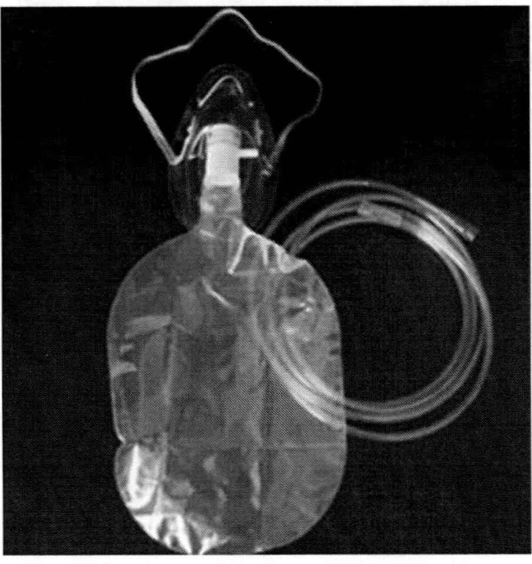

Partial Rebreathing Mask

5. **Non-Rebreathing Mask with reservoir**
   - It is similar to the partial rebreathing mask except it has a series of one-way valves preventing exhaled air from returning to the bag.

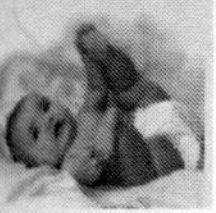

- High oxygen device.
- Delivers 95% Oxygen at 10-12 L/min.
- Two valves added to Rebreathing mask prevents entrainment of room air during inspiration.
- Retention of exhaled gases during expiration.

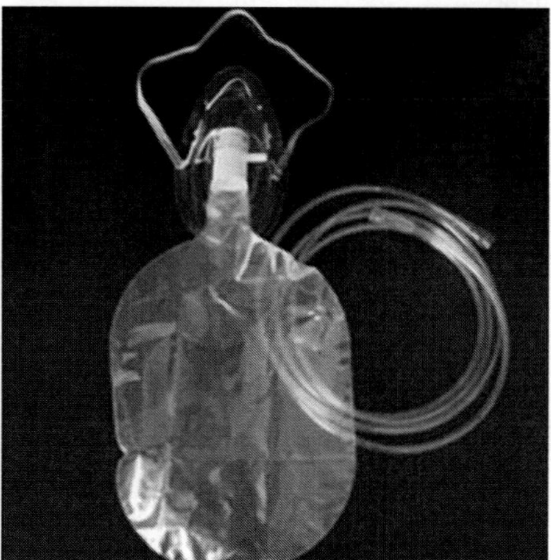

Non-Rebreathing Mask with reservoir

6. **Venturi mask**
   - It works on principle of venturi and delivers precise amount of O_2 as indicated on it with that flow of gas.
   - It prevent re breathing of CO_2.
   - Well tolerated by patient.
   - O_2 toxicity is less.

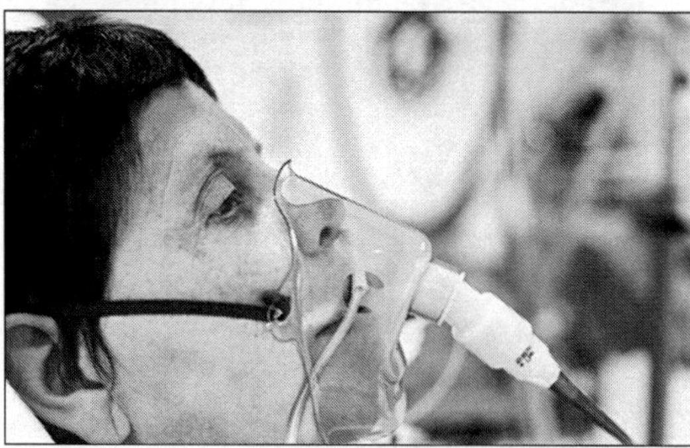

Venturi mask

7. **Oxygen tent**
   - An oxygen tent consists of a canopy placed over the head and shoulders or over the entire body of a patient to provide oxygen at a higher level than normal.
   - It is better for paediatrics patients and uncooperative patients.
   - 8 to 10 L/min of O_2 gives fio_2 50%.
   - O_2 therapy can be discontinued for feeding.
   - Danger of fire.

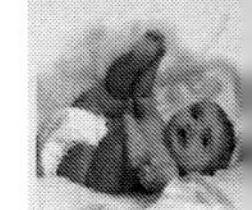

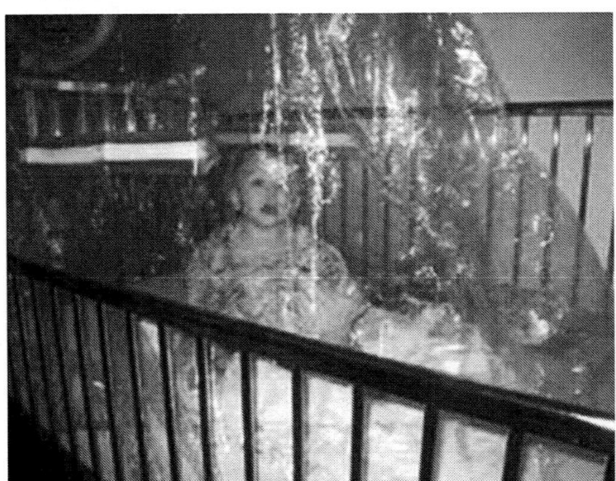

Oxygen tent

8. **Oxygen hood:** Transparent plexiglass hood of different sizes are used peadiatrics patients
   - 3 times/min of gas flow required.
   - O_2 therapy can be interrupted while giving feed.

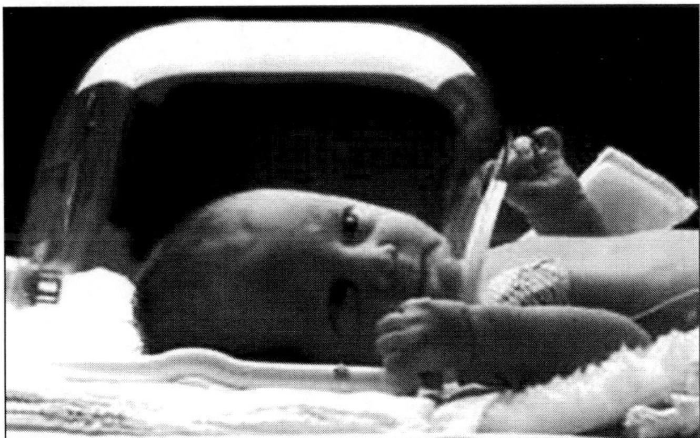

Oxygen hood

9. **Oxygen in incubator:** Child in incubator is given O_2 by this method.

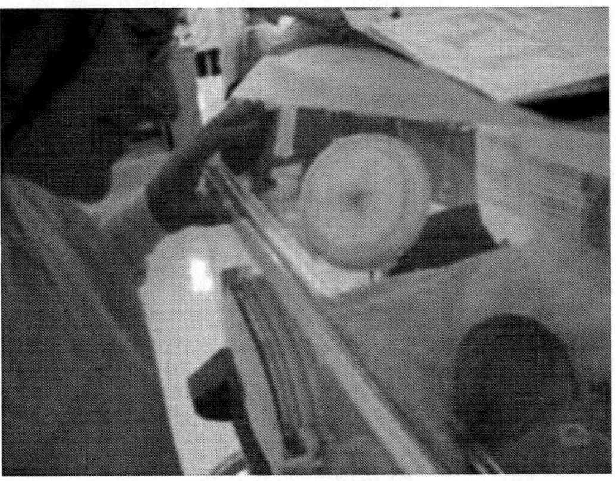

Oxygen in incubator

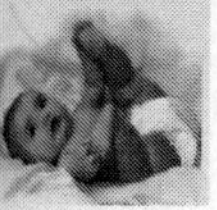

Invasive Devices

1. **Nasal Catheter:**
   - 8 to 14 FG catheter red rubber or portex are used.
   - Multiple holes should be made on patient end.
   - Should be well lubricated with anesthetic jelly before introduction.
   - Should reach just beyond nasopharynx.
   - Catheter should be changed every 8 to 10 hours.
   - With 6 L/min of oxygen fio$_2$ is 50%.
   - Can get blocked by secretions.

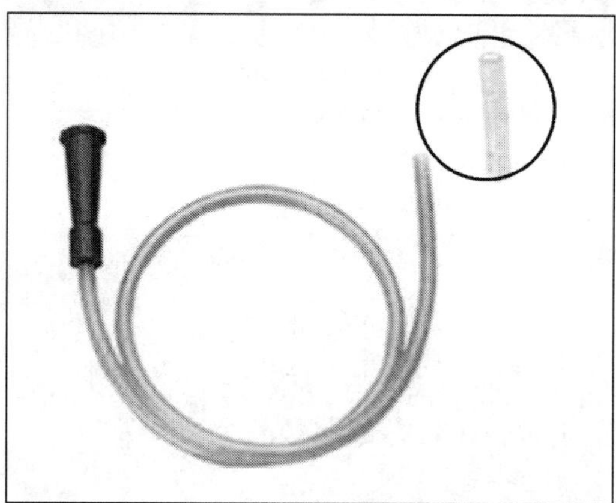

Nasal catheter

2. **Endotracheal Tube (Cuffed)**
   - Manufactured from siliconised non-toxic, non-irritant P.V.C.
   - Sensitive tube ensures tube patency for patient safety.
   - It softens at body temperature to conform to the anatomy of the respiratory tract.
   - Resistant inflation tube ensures patient safety during cuff inflation and deflation.

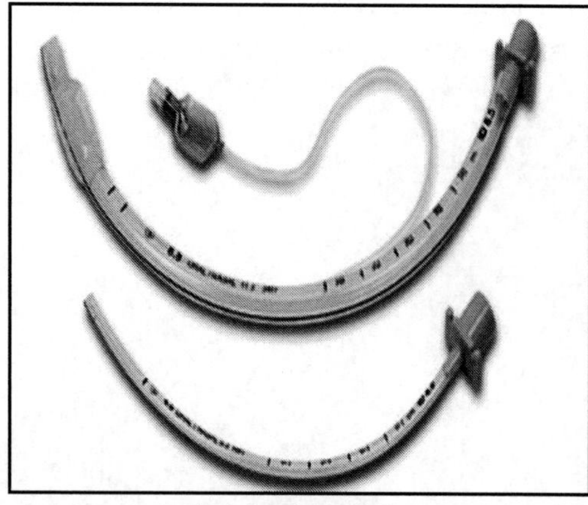

Endotracheal Tube

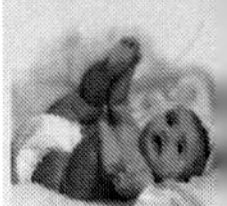

3. **Tracheostomy**
   - It is surgical procedure on the neck to open a direct airway through an incision in the trachea (the windpipe).
   - It is performed by surgeons. Both surgical and percutaneous techniques are now widely used.

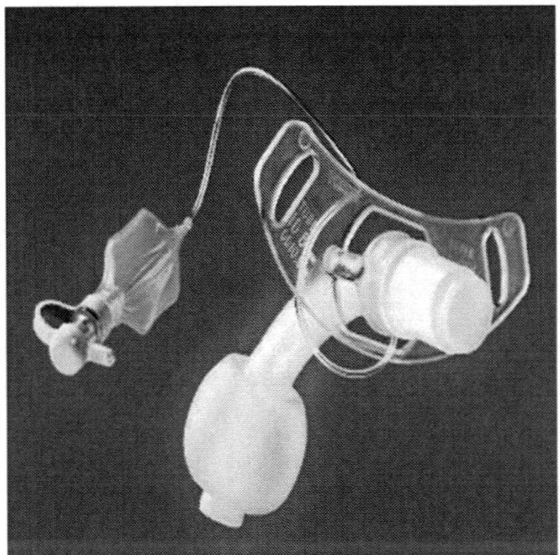

Tracheostomy

Other Important Oxygen Delivering Devices

The bag-valve mask:

- The bag-valve mask (BVM) is used for patients in critical condition who are either breathing extremely inefficiently, or not breathing at all (respiratory arrest).
- An oxygen reservoir bag is attached to a central cylindrical bag, attached to a valved mask that administers almost 100% concentration oxygen at 8-15 l/m.
- The central bag is squeezed manually to deliver a „breath" to the patient, or assist them in breathing by doing some of the work for the lungs.

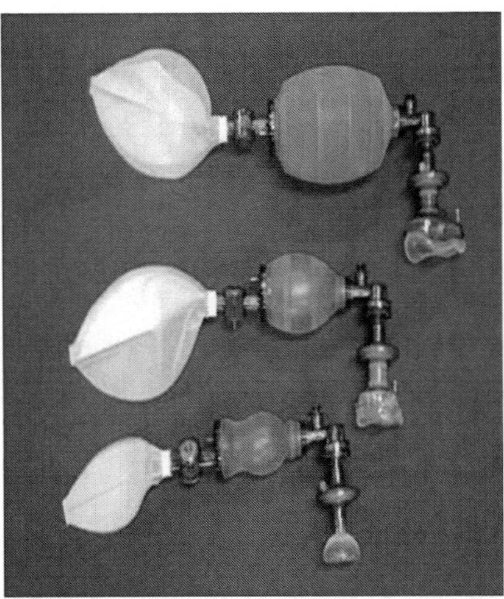

The bag-valve mask

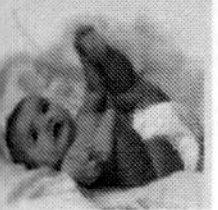

The pocket mask

- The pocket mask is a small device that can be used in emergency conditions.
- It is used by exhaling air into the mask.
- Exhaled air from the provider can provide up to 16% oxygen to the patient.

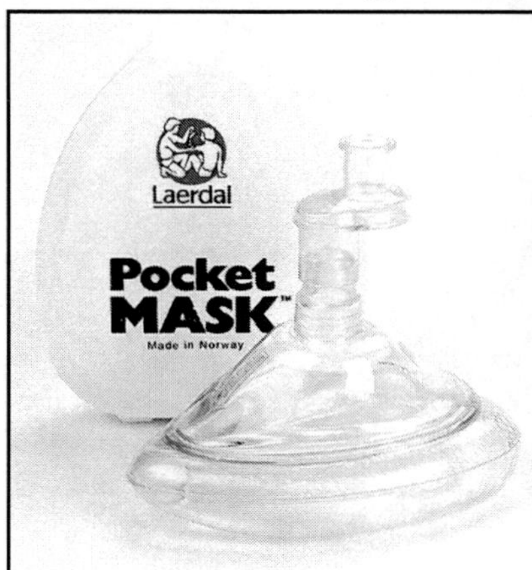

The pocket mask

Humidification

- Is recommended if more than 4 litres/min is delivered.
- Helps prevent drying of mucous membranes.
- Helps prevent the formation of tenacious sputum

Selection of Method of O_2 Therapy

Method is determined factor like

- Age and level of consciousness of patient.
- Level and cause of hypoxia.
- General condition of the patient.
- Facilities and expertise advice.
- Fio_2 required.

Procedure of oxygen therapy

1. Determine need for oxygen therapy in patient check physician order for rate, device to be used etc.
2. Perform an assessment of vital signs, level on consciousness, lab values etc.
3. Asses risk factor of oxygen therapy in patient and environment such as patient with hypoxia drive, faulty electrical connection etc.
4. Explain procedure to relatives and inform them how to cooperate.
5. Post no smoking sign on bed side of patient and explain them the dangers of smoking when oxygen is on flow.

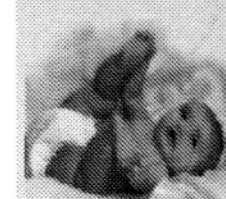

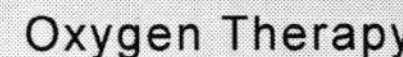

6. Wash hands.
7. Set up oxygen equipment and humidifier
   - Fill Humidifier up to level marked on it with sterile water.
   - Attach flow meter to source, set flow meter in off position.
   - Attach humidifier to base of flow meter.
   - Regulate flow meter to prescribed level.
   - Ensure proper functioning by checking for bubbles in humidifier or feeling oxygen at the outlet.
8. Place tips of cannula (in case nasal cannula is used) to patient's nares and adjust straps around the ears for snug fit the elastic band may be fixed behind head or under chin.
9. Inspect patient and equipment frequently for flow rate, clinical condition, level of water in humidifier etc.
10. Wash hands.
11. Document time, flow rate observation made on the patient.
12. Remove and clean the cannula with soap and water, dry and replace every 8 hrs. assess for at least 8 hrs.

Oxygen Safety

- If O_2 tank gets punctured, or valves break off, tank becomes a missile.
- O_2 supports combustion, causing fire to burn rapidly. Therefore no open flame or products that are combustible should be permitted when oxygen is in use.
- An explosion products that are combustible should not be permitted when oxygen is in use These include petroleum jelly, oils, and aerosol sprays. A spark from a cigarette, electric razor, or other electrical device could easily ignite oxygen-saturated hair or bedclothes around the patient.
- Don't lubricate the O_2 tank or gauges with petroleum products.
- Never roll a tank.
- Never store in heat or in a closed vehicle in the sun.
- No smoking or exposure to open flame around O_2.
- No tape on tank/gauges.
- O_2 reacts with some adhesives.
- Store tanks upright and secured.
- Place NO SMOKING sign near child.

Side Effects of Oxygen Therapy

- Oxygen has vasoconstrictive effects on the circulatory system, reducing peripheral circulation.
- In rare instances, hyperbaric oxygen therapy patients have had seizures.
- High levels of oxygen given to neonates causes blindness by promoting overgrowth of new blood vessels in the eye obstructing sight. This is retinopathy of prematurity (ROP).
- Administration of high levels of oxygen in patients with severe emphysema and high blood carbon dioxide reduces respiratory drive, which can precipitate respiratory failure and death.

CHAPTER 17

Nebulization

Introduction

Aerosol drug administration, also known as inhalation therapy, or in some cases, nebulized drug therapy, is the method by which drugs are dispersed into the lungs or bronchial airways in the form of tiny droplets – often bound to water, oxygen, or another gaseous substance. Drugs are generally delivered by two means. The first is via a device called a nebulizer. The nebulizer is a mechanical pump (of which there are many types) that produces a fine mist in which the drug is dispersed via an appropriate nebulizer-compatible face mask. This fine mist is inhaled deep into the lungs for maximum effect. The second method of delivery is via hand-held, nebulized aerosol device. These devices, also known as "puffers," use the effects of a pressurized gas to and disperse the drug into a fine mist or spray, which is then inhaled.

Definition

Nebulization is the process of delivering medication by a fine mist that is inhaled directly into the lungs. The jet medication nebulizer utilizes a high velocity has flow to generate particles from the prescribed solution. Either oxygen or compressed air powers the nebulizer.

Purposes

Aerosol administration of drugs is indicated in circumstance where rapid absorption and localized effects of the drug are required to produce the appropriate response.

- Asthmatic conditions
- Specific lung conditions that cause difficulty in breathing (emphysema, asthma, ARDS and other similar conditions that warrant and necessitate the use administration of drugs by this route.
- As routine postoperative intervention for those children with pulmonary edema

Articles Required

- Oxygen source (oxygen cylinder/wall oxygen outlet with flow meter).

A clean tray containing

- A face mask of appropriate size and oxygen tubing.

Nebulizer kit consisting of:

- Face mask/mouth piece.
- Nebulizer jar and nebulizer cap.
- Oxygen supply tubing.

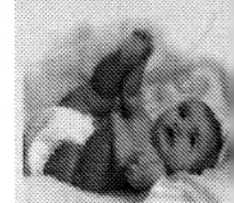

- Nebulizing solution (drug and normal saline for dilution).
- 2 ml and 5 ml syringes.
- Sputum mug.
- Nasal swab sticks.
- A bowl containing spirit swabs.
- A bowl containing normal saline swabs.
- A bowl containing dry cotton swabs.
- Kidney tray and paper bag.

Steps of the Procedure

1. Verify the instruction for nebulization.
2. Assemble the articles and bring them to the bedside.
3. Place the child in a comfortable, upright position that is greater than 45 degrees. This will enable maximum breathing efficiency. The comfort of the child should be ensured and maintained throughout the procedure.
4. Explain the procedure to the child and/or to the family and the child should be reassured if he is dyspneic and anxious and inhalation of the nebulized drug is assured.
5. Wash hands.
6. Prepare the neblulizer solution.
7. Clean the mask and the tubing, first with spirit swabs and then with normal saline swabs and dry them.
8. Put the medication in prescribed dilution into the nebulizer and keep it ready.
9. Clean the nostrils if dirty with the swab sticks.
10. When patient is comfortable and in a suitable position nebulization can be started.
11. Adjust the oxygen to a flow rate of 6-8 litres per minute or until a fine mist appears.
12. Or turn the nebulizer pump on.
13. Confirm that a steady mist is flowing from the mask or application device.
14. When a steady flow of mist is achieved, fit the mask or application device correctly to the patient's face or trachea (if applicable).
15. Instruct the child to breath in and out through the mouth slowly and completely.
16. While nebulizsation and delivery of drug is occurring, the patient should be monitored for signs of reaction to the drug and for improvement or deterioration in breathing patterns.
17. Monitor the child's oxygen saturation level throughout the procedure, if equipment is available.
18. Continue to have nebulizer dispense medication until all the medication has disappeared from the chamber.
19. Ask the child whether the medication has had a positive effect. If not, further advice or orders should be sought from the physician.
20. Record and report the procedure.
21. Dissemble the articles.

CHAPTER 18

Urinary Catheterization

Definition

It is the insertion of a catheter directly into the urinary bladder through the route of urethra.

Indications

The indications for urinary catheterization are:

- Conditions in which strict intake output records are to be maintained. For example renal.
- failure, CHF.
- Preoperatively.
- In case of urinary retention or incontinence e.g. neurogenic bladder.
- For collection of sterile urinary samples.

Articles Required

The articles required for urinary catheterization are:

- Foley's catheter of appropriate size.
- Urinary bag.
- 10 ml syringe filled with saline to fix the catheter.
- Pair of sterile gloves.
- Sterile drape sheet.
- Swabs and sponge holding forceps to provide perineal care.
- 1% savlon.
- Kidney tray to discard the waste papers.
- Skin friendly tape to secure the catheter, screen.

Steps of the Procedure

1. Assemble the required articles at patient's bedside.
2. Explain the procedure to the patient if possible or to the parents.
3. Give dorsal recumbent position to the patient.
4. Wash hands with soap and water.
5. Wear sterile gloves.

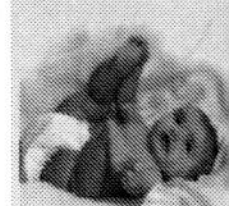

In females

1. Provide perineal care using 1% savlon.
2. Use single swab for single stroke.
3. Spread the sterile drape sheet exposing the perineal area.
4. Lubricate the tip of the catheter.
5. Use nondominant hand to separate the majors.
6. Insert the catheter gently into the urinary meatus.
7. Advance the catheter till urine pours out.
8. At that point advance the catheter about 1-2 inches more.
9. Fix the catheter with the help of normal saline, Inflate the balloon.
10. Attach the foley's to the urinary bag.
11. Lastly fix the catheter to the thigh with the help of a skin friendly tape.

In males

1. Clean the fore skin around meatus with 1% savlon.
2. Hold the penis in nondominant hand.
3. With other hand retract the fore skin and gently insert the catheter into urinary meatus.
4. Advance the catheter until urine comes.
5. At this point insert the catheter 1-2 inches more.
6. Fix the catheter with the help of normal saline to inflate the balloon.
7. Attach the catheter to the urinary bag and secure to catheter with tape.

After Care

A. Patient

- Before leaving ensure that patient is in comfortable position.

B. Articles

- Terminate the procedure properly.
- Replace the articles after washing.

CHAPTER 19

Enema

Introduction

Enema are used to help relieve impacted bowel movements. Children may be prescribed enema by a doctor after surgery or if they have been constipated or are not having regular bowel movements.

Definition

Administration of fluid into the lower bowel through the rectum for the purpose of cleansing or to introduce medication is known as enema.

Purpose

- To simulate defecation
- To treat constipation.
- To soften the hard fecal matter.
- To administer medication.
- To protect and soothen mucus membrane of the intestine.
- To destroy intestinal parasites.
- To relieve gaseous distension.
- To administer fluid and nutrients.
- To relieve inflammation.
- To introduce peristalsis.
- To reduce temperature.
- To establish regular bowel function.

General Instruction

- The appropriate size catheter or rectal tube need to be used. For giving a cleansing enema (12 Fr for an infant and no 14 to 18 Fr for school age child.)
- The rectal tube need to be smooth and flexible.
- The rectal tube is lubricated with a water soluble lubricant.
- The temperature of the solutions needs to be adjusted according to the purpose of enema.
- The amount of solution to be administered depends upon the type of enema and the age and size of the person. For giving evacuant enema 250 to 500 ml for a child and 250 ml or less for an infant can be used.

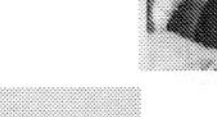

- When an enema is administered the patient usually assumes a left lateral position.
- The distance to which the tube is inserted depends upon the age and size of the patient. For children 2.5 to 3.75 cm.
- Height of the enema can should be adjusted to regulate the flow of solution.
- To retain the solution, the nurse can press the baby's buttocks together.
- Prevent air from entering the rectum.

Preliminary Assessment

- Check the diagnosis.
- Check the date and type of surgery.
- Check the nature of enema ordered.
- Check for any lesions on the rectal and perineal area.

Articles Required

A tray containing

- Enema can, tubing, screw.
- Clamp.
- Rectal catheter.
- Mackintosh and towel.
- Water soluble jelly/enema pouch/proctoclysis pouch.
- Rag pieces.
- Hot and cold water in jugs.
- Soap jelly.
- Ounce glass.
- Kidney tray.
- Bed pan.
- Clean linen.
- I/V stand.
- Screen.

Preparation of Patient and Environment

- Explain procedure to the child if old enough if not, then to parents.
- Provide privacy with Curtains/Screen.
- Cover patient with sheet.
- Remove back rest and pillows.
- Place mackintosh and towel under patient's buttock.
- Place patient in left lateral position.

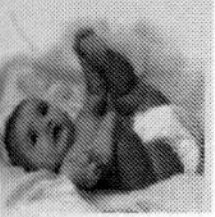

- Keep bed pan under bed.
- Adjust I/V pole to required height.
- Remove bottom garments.

Steps of the Procedure

1. Wash hands.
2. Attach tubing to the enema can and clamp the tube.
3. Prepare the solution at the required temperature.
4. Hang the can with the solution on the stand and adjust the height at 45 cm.
5. Attach a rectal tube to the tubing. Loosen the screw clamp and let a small amount of fluid to run into the kidney tray.
6. Lubricate the tip of the rectal tube about 2 or 4 inches from the tip/ tip of the enema pouch.
7. Separate the patient's buttocks to visualize the anus clearly and insert the tip 8 to 10 cm inside the anal canal.
8. Hold the enema tube in place while releasing the pressure on the tube and let the fluid run in.
9. Stop the procedure if the patient develops discomfort.
10. Clamp the tubing, gently remove the rectal tube by pulling it through 3 to 4 layers of rag pieces, gauze pieces.
11. Discard the rag pieces in the paper bag. Detach the rectal tube and place it in the kidney tray.

After Care of the Patient and Articles

- Encourage the patient to retain the fluid for 10 to 15 min.
- Turn the patient on back and assist him onto toilet help the child to defecate in his/her natural posture.
- Take all articles to the utility room. Disinfect the rectal tube, clean it, boil it and store it in its proper place.
- Wash hands.
- Return to bedside and evaluate patient's condition.
- Send the specimen if any to the laboratory.

SUPPOSITORY

Introduction

It acts as a local irritant which stimulates excretion by absorbing in the mucosa, while others act directly on the nerve endings and stimulate peristalsis.

Definition

Suppositories are solid, cone shaped or oval shaped masses that melt at body temperature.

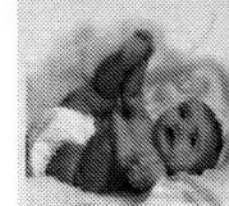

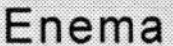

Articles Required

- Suppository.
- Gloves.
- Kidney Tray.
- Mackintosh.
- Drawsheet.
- Bedpan.

Steps of the Procedure

1. Before introducing suppository, explain procedure to the child if old enough.
2. Patient is placed in a comfortable position, usually left lateral position.
3. Suppository is removed from its package and hold it in the right hand between the two fingers.
4. Separating the buttocks with the left hand insert the suppository into the anus.
5. Once it has passed the external sphincter, advance it beyond the internal sphincter, pushing it with index finger and in infants with little finger.
6. Patient should be instructed to retain the suppository as long as it is comfortable for about 20 to 30 minutes or even longer.

CHAPTER 20

Care of Baby Under Phototherapy

Introduction

Neonatal jaundice is a common condition among newborn babies and phototherapy is the effective and reliable method of its management.

Definition

Phototherapy is the procedure in which the baby is exposed to visible lights which causes the photo-oxidation and photo isomerization of bilirubin into water soluble, colorless form of bilirubin.

For phototherapy to be effective, bilirubin needs to be present in skin so there is no role of prophylactic phototherapy. It acts by several ways:

1. **Configurational Isomerization:** Here the z-isomers of bilirubin are converted into e-isomers. the reaction is instantaneous upon exposure to light but reversible as bilirubin reaches into bile duct. since this is excreted from body this is not a major mechanism for decrease in stb.
2. **Structural Isomerization:** This is an irreversible reaction to convert bilirubin into lumirubin. the reaction is directly proportional to the dose of phototherapy. this product forms 2-6% of stb which is rapidly excreted from body thus mainly responsible for phototherapy induced decline in stb.
3. **Photo oxidation:** This is a minor reaction, photo products are excreted in urine.

Procedure of Phototherapy

1. Undress the baby completely.
2. The baby's eyes are shielded by an opaque mask to prevent exposure to the light as phototherapy can cause damage to photoreceptors in the retina.
3. The eye shield should be properly sized and correctly positioned to cover the eye completely but prevent any occlusion of the nares.
4. The baby's eyelids are closed before the mask is applied, because the corneas may become excoriated if they come in contact with the dressing.
5. On each nursing shift the eyes are checked for evidence of discharge, excessive pressure on the lids or corneal irritation. Give daily eye care to baby.
6. Eye shields are removed during feedings, which provide the opportunity to provide visual and sensory stimulation.
7. During breastfeeding switch off the photo therapy unit.
8. Provide frequent breast feeding (approx. after 2 hours).

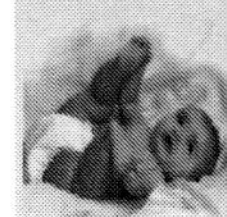

9. Turn the baby after each feed to expose maximum surface area of baby to light.
10. Keep baby at a distance of 45 cm from the light source. The distance can be reduced to 15-20 cm to provide more effective or intensive phototherapy.
11. A special light - permeable photo therapy diaper, or bikini diaper fashioned with a face mask may be used to cover the genitalia and buttocks.
12. Keep diaper area dry and clean because skin in this area is prone to break down.
13. Babies who are in an open crib must have a protective plexiglas shield between them and the fluorescent light to minimize the amount of un desirable ultraviolet light reaching their skin and to protect them from accidental bulb breakage.
14. Monitor temperature every two to four hour or more frequently if fluctuation in temperature is noted.
15. Maintaining the baby in a flexed position with rolled blankets along the sides of the body helps maintain heat and provides comfort.
16. Maintain thermoneutrality - measure incubator or isolate temperature as well as infant's light affects the ambient temperature.
17. Do not expose the thermistor probe to the light without the probe's being covered with opaque tape
18. Adequate fluid intake should be provided either orally or intravenously, vasodilation increases the insensible water loss and there is excess stool loss from occasional diarrhea, keep urine specific gravity below 1.015. (Breastfeeding or 10-20% extra fluids are provided).
19. Ensure that the baby passes adequate urine (6-8 times per day).
20. Weight is taken at least once a day.
21. Ensure that serum bilirubin levels are obtained as prescribed. The diminishing icterus, i.e. the lowering of unconjugated bilirubin from cutaneous tissue does not reflect the serum bilirubin concentration.
22. Discontinue photo therapy when serum bilirubin returns to a safe value as per unit protocol.
23. Monitor clinically for rebound bilirubin rise within 24 hours after stopping phototherapy for babies with hemolytic disorders.
24. Accurate charting is another important nursing responsibility that includes:
    - time that photo therapy is started and stopped.
    - proper shielding of the eyes, and covering of the testes (genitals).
    - type of fluorescent lamp (by manufacture).
    - number of lamps.
    - distance between surface of lamps and infant (should be not less than 45 cms).
    - use of photo therapy in combination with an incubator or open bassinet.
    - photometer measurement of light intensity.
    - occurrence of side effect.
    - length of time the bulbs have been used.
    - the effectiveness of light of the wave length decreases after 800 hours, of use; thus bulbs should be changed at the correct time. A record of hours of use is essential.

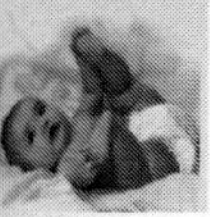

- record vital signs every 2 hourly.
- maintain feeding chart, weight chart, regularly.
- serum bilirubin is monitored at least every 12 hours.
- record weight daily.

Complications of Phototherapy

The predominant side effects of phototherapy are as following:

a. Lethargy.

b. Loose green stool(due to accelerated intestinal transit time).

c. Increased insensible water loss- provide more frequent extra breastfeeding.

d. Dark Urine.

e. Temperature elevation.

f. Skin changes - greenish colour, rash due to capillary dilation - skin rashes - no need to discontinue photo therapy.

g. Increased metabolic rate, dehydration, and electrolyte disturbances such as hypocalcemia.

h. Retina damage: prevented by shielding the eyes.

i. Hypo or hyperthermia: Monitor temperature frequently.

j. Bronze-baby syndrome - in which the serum, urine and skin turn grayish brown several hours after the infant is placed under the light. This reaction is probably caused by retention of a bilirubin break down product of phototherapy, possibly copper porphyrin. The syndrome almost always occurs in infants who have elevated conjugated hyperbilirubinemia and some degree of cholestasis. The browning generally resolves following discontinuation of phototherapy.

k. Photo therapy has been shown to affect short terms behavior of the term infant, which has been attributed to maternal separation. This least discussed and often overlooked aspect, is the most common side effect, so one should encourage the mother to breastfeed and interact with her baby regularly during phototherapy.

Caution

1. Do not use photo therapy without trying to find the cause of Jaundice.
2. Photo therapy results in dehydration and iatrogenic hyperthermia/hypothermia.
3. Blue light may interfere with monitoring of cyanosis. Blue light cause nausea, giddiness and headache which may affect/disturb the staff.
4. In direct hyperbilirubinemia, photo therapy results in Bronze baby syndromes (green colour).
5. Nurse should wear sun glass and cover the hair with a cap or bandana, when caring for an infant under blue light for her own protection.
6. If the nurses skin is sensitive to the lights a screening substance may be used to prevent tanning of exposed area.

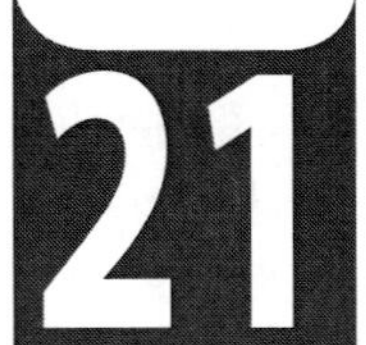

Care of Ostomy and Colostomy

Introduction

Ostomy is a surgical procedure in which an opening is made through the skin directly into a hollow organ of the body. A stoma is an artificial opening created to the surface of the body. Colostomy (colon), ileostomy (ileum), cystostomy (urinary bladder), nephrostomy (kidney), ureterostomy (ureter) are some of the common ostomies we come across according to the underlying pathology of the patient.

Here we will discuss colostomy, the commonest of all which we come across in our clinical practice.

Colostomy Care

Colostomy refers to a surgical procedure where a portion of the large intestine is brought through the abdominal wall through which stool is to be excreted. The surface of the stoma is actually the lining of the intestine, usually appearing moist and pink. Colostomy may be temporary or permanent according to the underlying pathology. Colostomy care refers to the procedure of cleaning the stoma intermittently along with the surrounding skin in order to keep it clean, healthy and functional.

Indications of Colostomy

Children may require colostomy for various health problems

- Imperforate anus in infants.
- Necrotising enterocolitis.
- Hirschsprung's disease.

Types of colostomy

1. **End colostomy:** The functioning end of the intestine (the section of bowel that remains connected to the upper gastrointestinal tract) is brought out onto the surface of the abdomen, forming the stoma by cuffing the intestine back on itself and suturing the end to the skin. The distal portion of bowel (now connected only to the rectum) may be removed or sutured closed and left in the abdomen. An end colostomy is usually a permanent ostomy, resulting from trauma, cancer or another pathological condition.
2. **Double-barrel colostomy:** This colostomy involves the creation of two separate stomas on the abdominal wall. The proximal stoma is the functional end that is connected to the upper gastrointestinal tract and will drain stool. The distal stoma, connected to the rectum and also called a mucous fistula, drains small amounts of mucus material. This is most often a temporary colostomy performed to rest an area of bowel, and to be closed later.

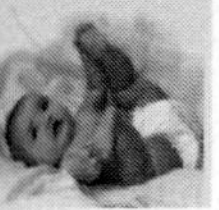

3. **Loop colostomy:** This colosotmy is created by bringing a loop of bowel through an incision in the abdominal wall. The loop is held in place outside the abdomen by a plastic rod slipped beneath it. An incision is made in the abdomen to allow the passage of stool through the loop colostomy. The supporting rod is removed approximately 7-10 days after surgery, when healing has occurred that will prevent the loop bowel from retracting into the abdomen. A loop colosotmy is most often performed for creation of a temporary stoma to divert stool away from an area of intestine that has been blocked or ruptured.

CARE OF COLOSTOMY

Introduction

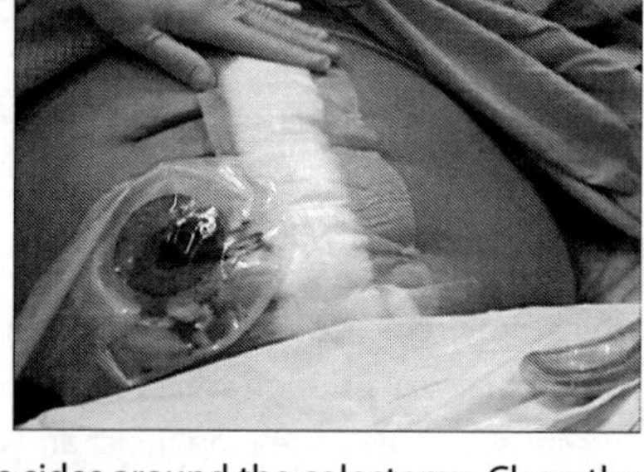

1. Remove the soiled dressing and discard into the polythene bag/newspaper.
2. Wash your hands thoroughly with soap and water.
3. Take the cotton swab; soak in the water; squeeze and clean the stomal opening with the swab when it is dirty and discard it in the polythene bag/newspaper.
4. Take another cotton swab; soak in the water, squeeze and clean the pericolostomy skin. Use two swabs to clean both the sides around the colostomy. Clean the pericolostomy skin with dry swabs, once it is completely dry leave it.
5. Take some siloderm ointment/Vaseline/coconut oil/sarson oil/zinc oxide on the tip of your finger.
6. Apply it around the stoma.
7. Cover the colostomy with a small piece of soft cloth soaked in coconut oil then place cotton or small dressing on the stoma. Cotton should be used for newborns during first few days because their skin is very delicate.
8. Support the dressing by tying the long cloth bandage around the baby's tummy and wash your hands.

The skin around the colostomy is constantly in touch with intestinal juices which causes excoriation. Application of siloderm protects the skin from excoriation caused by intestinal juices and injury. The skin around the colostomy should be cleaned every time the dressing is changed.

COLOSTOMY BAG AND ITS USE

Introduction

Plastic colostomy bags are available in the market, which can be applied on the colostomy stoma. The feces can be collected in the bag. Each bag costs about 150 rupees and lasts for 10-15 days and the other costing about 40 rupees can be used for one day.

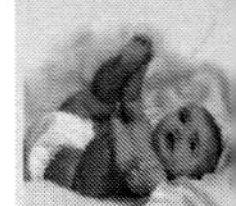

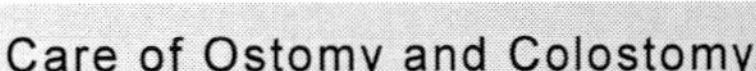

APPLICATION OF BAG ON STOMA

Introduction

1. Gently remove the soiled dressing or bag. Wash hands thoroughly with soap and water. Clean stoma and peri-colostomy skin.
2. Measure the size of the stoma with a measuring guide.
3. Cut the wafer with scissor according to the size of the stoma.
4. Take some siloderm ointment on the tip of your finger and apply around the stoma.
5. Apply the colostomy bag around stoma and secure the wafer with adhesive tape.
6. Check the bag for air leak by gently pressing the bag. The bag should be changed when filled with fecal matter.

CHAPTER 22

Bowel Wash

Introduction

Regular elimination of bowel waste products is essential for normal body functioning. Alterations in elimination can cause problems with the gastrointestinal and other body systems.

Definition

Bowel wash is the, introduction of isotonic fluid into the upper bowel segment through the rectum for the purpose of cleansing and removal of waste.

Purpose of Bowel Wash

Therapeutic purposes to cleanse the bowel.

- Hepatic encephalopathy
- Hirsch sprung's disease.
- GI tract poisoning.
- Management of fecal incontinence.

General instructions for giving bowel wash

- The appropriate size catheter or rectal tube need to be used. 12 Fr catheter for an infant and number 14 to 18 Fr for the school age child.
- The rectal tube need to be smooth and flexible.
- The rectal tube is lubricated with a water soluble lubricant.
- The amount of the solution to be administered depends on the age of the child. Normally, 100 ml of normal saline is used for children.
- For children the tube is inserted up to 2.5 to 3.5 inch. If any obstruction is encountered it should be withdrawn and reported.
- The height of the enema can should be above 45 cm.

Articles Required

A tray containing

- 14-18 no red rubber flatus tube for a 4-5 year old child.
- Enema can (if a plastic nozzle is attached to the tubing which can directly be inserted in the anus then a rubber flatus tube is not required).

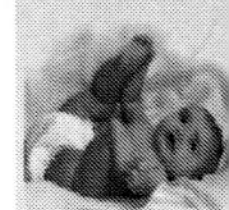

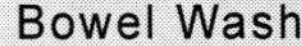

- Luke warm water or isotonic solution like normal saline.
- Lubricating jelly.
- Mackintosh with paper lining.
- Gauze pieces or cotton swabs to separate the buttocks.
- Some cotton pads to wipe the child.
- Gloves.
- Bed pan.

Points to Remember

The child should be explained the purpose for which bowel wash is given.

Steps of the Procedure

1. Assemble all articles at the bed side.
2. Make the child lie in side lateral position at one edge of the bed, spread the mackintosh with paper lining underneath.
3. Fill the enema can with water or solution.
4. Attach the red rubber flatus tube to the tubing of enema can and fold the tube so that water does not spill or (if there is clamp on the nozzle of the enema can, close it) make the tubings air free.
5. Wear gloves.
6. Lubricate the tip of the red rubber tube or plastic nozzle by applying lubricating jelly.
7. Gently insert the red rubber tube or the plastic nozzle in the anus of the child. (approx 2-3 inch inside). Separate the buttocks using the gauze pieces or cotton swabs.
8. Elevate the enema can so that water flows to the rectum. Open the clamp of the nozzle or unfold the tubing.
9. Disconnect the connection of the enema can and hold the end of the rubber catheter in the bed pan for back flow.
10. Repeat the procedure, till the back flow is clear.
11. Wipe and clean the child.
12. Make the child comfortable.
13. Wash the tubing with soap and water, replace the enema can and articles. Wash your hands with soap.
14. Complete the recordings. Recordings include – the date, time, type of solution used for bowel wash and the type of back flow. Also if there is any complication like, obstruction etc. mention it. At last put your initials.

Conclusion

Bowel wash though seems to be bit tedious procedure, if done systematically can prove to be of great therapeutic value.

CHAPTER 23

Handwashing

Definition

It is the most important means of preventing nosocomial infections. It is very simple and cheap.

Handwashing Norm

- 2 minutes handwashing (6 steps) to be done before entering the unit.
- 20 seconds handwashing to be done before and after touching babies.

Golden Rules

Six Steps of Handwashing

1. Step 1 – Palm and Finger.
2. Step 2 – Back of Hands.
3. Step 3 – Finger and Knuckles.
4. Step 4 – Thumbs.
5. Step 5 – Finger Tips.
6. Step 6 – Wrists and Forearms.

Once you have washed your hands, do not touch anything, till you carry out the required job.

- Keep elbows always dependent, i.e. at a lower level than your hands.
- Close the tap with elbow.
- Dry hand using single – use sterile napkin or autoclaved newspaper pieces.
- Discard napkin in the bin kept for the purpose, put newspaper pieces in the black bucket.
- Do not keep long or polished nails.

CHAPTER 24

Management of Breastfeeding

Introduction

The best milk for newborn baby is unquestionably breast milk. All healthy normal weight babies (≥ 2500 g) must be exclusively breastfeed till the age of 6 months.

Breastfeeding is beneficial for the health of baby as well as the mother and it benefits the whole family, emotionally and economically.

Breastfeeding gives children the best start in life. It is estimated that over one million children die each year for diarrhea, respiratory and other infection because they are not adequately breastfed. Breastfeeding also helps to protect mother's health.

Management

Step 1: Preparing the infant and the mother

- Ensure that the infant is clinically stable.
- Ensure that infant is alert.
- Make sure that the mother is comfortable and relaxed.
- Make her sit down in a comfortable and convenient position.

Step 2: Demonstrate various positions for breastfeeding a baby

- Underarm position
- Using the opposite arm.
- Mother in lying down position.

Step 3: Demonstrate the four key points in position

- Baby's head and body should be straight.
- Baby's face should face mother's breast.
- Baby's body should be close to her body.
- Mother should support the baby's whole body.

Step 4: Show the mother how to support her breast with the other hand

Explain the mother that she should

- Put her fingers below her breast.
- Use her first finger to support the breast.

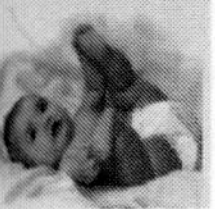

- Put her thumb above the areola helping to shape the breast.
- Not to keep her fingers near the nipple.

Step 5: Showing the mother how to help the baby to attach

Ask the mother to

- Express a little milk on to her nipple.
- Touch the baby's lips with her nipple.
- Wait until the baby's mouth is opening wide, and the tongue is down and forward.
- Move the baby quickly onto her breast, aiming the nipple towards the baby's palate and his lower lip well below the nipple.

Step 6: Look for signs of good attachment

The four key signs of good attachment are:

- More areola is visible above the baby's mouth than below it.
- Baby's mouth is wide open.
- Baby's lower lip is turned outwards.
- Baby's chin is touching the breast.

Step 7: Assess if the infant is suckling and swallowing effectively

Effective suckling

- Infant takes several deep sucks followed by swallowing and then pauses.
- Ineffective suckling.
- Infant suckles for a short time but tires out and is unable to continue for long enough.
- Frequency of breastfeeding.
- A healthy newborn baby can be breastfeed on demand, i.e. whenever the baby cries for feeds.
- The usual time interval between each feed is about 2 to 3 hours.
- They should feed their babies at least 8-10 times in 24 hours.
- They should not omit any night feeds.

Assessing the adequacy of breastfeeding

- Passes urine 6-8 times in 24 hours.
- Goes to sleep for 2-3 hours after the feeds.
- Gains weight @ 10-15 gm/kg/day.
- Crosses birth weight by 2 weeks.

SECTION 2

Advanced Nursing Procedures

CHAPTER 25

Newborn Assessment

Introduction

Once an baby is born he/she requires a thorough skilled observation and examination to ensure a satisfactory adjustment to the extrauterine life. The physical assessment represents a screening procedure to identify the likelihood of any pathology in a specific system to identify any deviation or abnormality in that system.

During physical assessment it is essential that the baby should not be disturbed so that a successful examination can be conducted.

Definition

It is detailed and systematic whole body examination of a stabilized newborn during early hours of life.

Purpose

- To determine the normalcy of different body systems for a healthy adaptation to extrauterine life.
- To detect significant medical problems for immediate management.
- To determine the cause and the extent of disease.
- To detect any congenital abnormality present for early management.

First examination: At birth look for- respiration, heart rate, color, neuromuscular activity, maturity, gestational age.

Second examination: A thorough & detailed one within 24 hours after birth.

Third examination: At the time of discharge from the health facility.

General Instructions

1. Examination should be done in a warm thermo neutral environment.
2. Examining hands must be thoroughly washed & made warm before examination.

Methods

Inspection

- Visual examination of the body is called inspection.

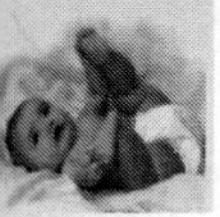

Palpation

- It is the feeling of the body or a part with the hands to note the size and positions of the organs.

Percussion

- It is the examination by tapping with the fingers on the body to determine the condition of the internal organs by the sound that are produced.

Auscultation

- It is the listening to sound within the body with the aid of the stethoscope.

Manipulation

- It is the moving of a part of the body to note its flexibility.

Testing of reflexes

- Testing reflexes is an important part of the neurological examination.

Articles Required

- Stethoscope.
- TPR Tray.
- Measuring Tape.
- Torch.
- Weighing machine.
- Soft Rubber Catheter.
- Draw sheet.
- Clean Gloves.

Steps of the Procedure

1. Wash hands thoroughly and wear gloves.
2. Uncover the baby and note general appearance. For normal baby findings include; body symmetrical and cylindrical in contour, head large in proportion to body, narrow chest, protruding abdomen and small hips.
3. Take head and body measurements. Normal measurements are; head circumference 33-35cm, chest circumference 30-33cm, crown rump length 34-35cm and crown heel length 48-52cm.
4. Assess skin, note the color of skin especially around mouth and finger nail beds. Normal skin is smooth, soft, elastic, warm and moist. The skin is pink, nail beds are blue,color of palms and nail beds will improve with activity.
5. Note any vascular nevi, milia, Mongolian spots or trauma marks on head, neck or body.
6. Assess head, examine head for symmetry, caput, cephalhematoma. Swelling on scalp from pressure of cervix indicates caput succedaneum. Subperiosteal bleeding, which does not cross suture line

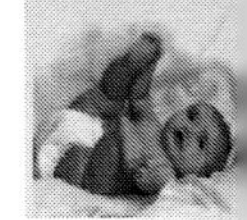

indicates cephalhematoma. Depressed fontanelle indicates dehydration and bulging fontanelle indicates increased intracranial pressure.

7. Assess face, observe symmetry of infant's face, note any characteristic features like flattened nose, folds below eyes, upturned nose etc. Asymmetry is usually related to damage to the facial nerve and becomes obvious when infant cries.
8. Assess eyes, examine the baby's eyes for response to light, puffiness, disc harge,opacity or conjuctival hemorrhage. Normally the eyes are gray, blue or brown in color. Infants will close their eyes in response to light, puffiness is common after forceps delivery, subconjuctival hemorrhage occurs due to pressure on fetal head during delivery, opacity suggest cataract formation, ptosis of eyelid suggest nerve damage.
9. Assess ears, examine the ears for firm and cartilaginous, presence of ear canal and hearing, location on head. Ear lobes are firm and cartilaginous in mature or term babies, deformed ear lobes with upper margin of the pinna rolled down and thickened are seen in down syndrome. Low set ears are seen in trisomy 15 and 18.
10. Assess mouth, examine the mouth and note the presence of any cleft lip or palate, Epstein pearls, asymmetry when crying, nasal teeth, macroglossia, pooling of saliva. Asymmetry of the mouth when open indicates facial nerve paralysis, pooling of saliva is sign of trachea-esophageal fistula/atresia. Macroglossia is seen in down syndrome.
11. Assess neck, examine neck for free movements, neck webbed on shoulders, extended arms on one side (shoulder dystocia), tightness of muscles on one side. Neck webbed on shoulders is seen in down's syndrome and turner's syndrome. Extension of one arm indicates clavicle fracture or damage to brachial nerve. Tightness of neck muscles is a sign of torticollis.
12. Assess chest, examine the chest for shape and movement of breathing, respiratory pattern, grunting sound on expiration, retraction on inspiration, heart rate, clavicles palpable on both sides. Quiet and free respiration at the rate of 40-60/min is normal. Grunting indicates respiratory distress. Clavicles clearly palpable if fracture is present.
13. Assess abdomen, observe the shape of abdomen and note shape, umbilical cord stump for presence of three vessels, any mass, bowel sounds, passage of meconium. Normal abdomen should be round and protruding, small scaphoid abdomen indicate diaphragmatic hernia. If three vessels are not found in umbilical cord stump congenital malformation should be suspected, mass may indicate umbilical or inguinal hernia, passage of meconium indicate patent anus.
14. Assess genitalia: Male; examine if foreskin covers the glans penis, uretheral meatus opens at tip of the penis and testicles are palpable in the scrotum bilaterally. Normally foreskin covers glans penis, deviation indicates hypospadias or epispadias, if testicles are not palpable, undescended testicles should be investigated. In case of female; labia minora is prominent and is not covered by labia majora, edematous genitalia, vaginal discharge or pseudomensuration. Edema is normal and vaginal discharge is normal response to maternal hormones.
15. Assess back, hold the newborn in prone position and examine back to evaluate spine, note presence of any dimple in coccygeal area, sinus opening or spina bifida, tufts of hair.

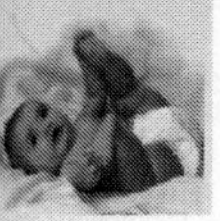

16. Assess anus, verify the presence of a perforate anus by inserting a soft rubber catheter gently into rectum (if newborn passes meconium earlier patency need not to be checked). Absence of meconium indicates imperforate anus.
17. Assess the upper extremities; note the proportion to the rest of body, symmetry and spontaneous movement of arms and hands, check if fingers show webbing, polydactylism or syndactylism, any skin tags.
18. Assess lower extremities, check for symmetry and length, range of motion, proportion to rest of body, symmetry of creases of legs and buttocks, assess feet for presence of club foot.
19. Inform parents about baby's condition and wellbeing.
20. Record findings in the newborn assessment record.

CHAPTER 26

Care of Child in Incubator

Introduction

Incubators are apparatus for maintaining optimal conditions of high risk preterm neonates. It is essential to provide an ideal micro-environment.

The main functions of incubators are isolation, maintenance of thermo neutral ambient temperature, desired humidity & administration of oxygen. It is desirable to nurse extremely low birth weight stable babies in incubator.

Thus an incubator is an apparatus used to maintain environmental conditions suitable for a neonate (newborn baby). It is used in preterm births or for some ill full-term babies.

Definition

Incubator can be defined as a microenvironment meant for placing newborns that are at high-risk for maintenance of body temperature.

Indications: The main indications for keeping baby in Incubator are:

- Premature Babies
- Hypothermia

Purposes

- To maintain temperature.
- To provide humidity.
- To administer oxygen.
- For observation of baby.
- To prevent infection.

Types of Incubator

- Portable.
- Standard.

Parts of Incubator

1. Deck.
2. Mattress which is enclosed by a clear plastic canopy.
3. Air intake pipe.

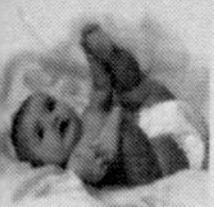

4. Micro filter assembly.
5. Oxygen Inlet.
6. Thermostat.
7. Calibrated dial.
8. Arm ports.
9. **Hood:** Single walled rectangular hood. The hood has larger door to aid in placing or removing baby from incubator. There are four ports for better access during small procedures, inlet for IV tubes, probes etc.
10. **Control Panel:** Heater, blower & electronics.
11. **Lower Unit:** This consists of control box; touch sensor, front panel with display, humidifier, air ducts & filters. The following are displayed on front of panel:
    - Air temperature.
    - Patient temperature.
    - Control temperature.
12. **Cabinet:** This provides support for hood, canopy & lower unit. It houses main switch, fuse & power connector. The cabinet has 3 drawers for storage purpose.
13. **Humidity Percentage:** Air is circulated by configural blower. Fresh air enters through air filters located at the edge of incubator. Fresh air is mixed with circulating air from incubator canopy & passed over heater & humidifier. Temperature inside incubator is maintained by sensor placed on hood. Thus, heated air flow maintains surroundings of infant at desired temperature.

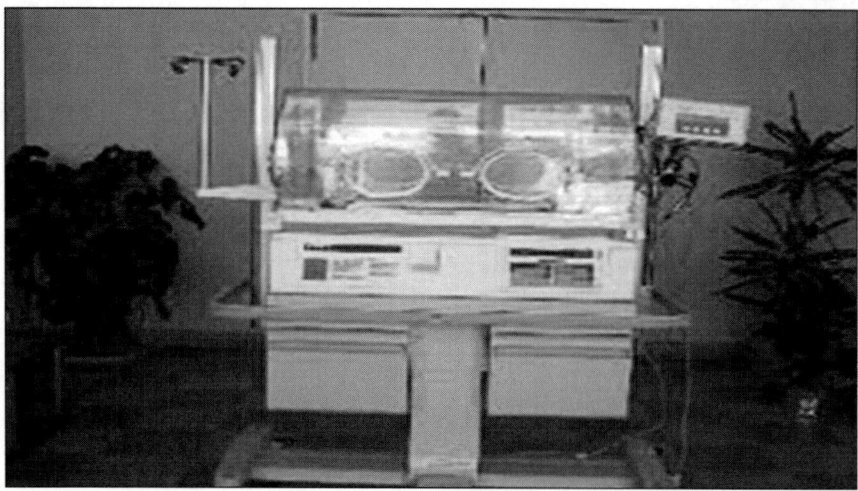

Incubator

Nursing Care of Child in Incubator

1. Identify the premature, weak or sick baby who needs to be nursed in an incubator.
2. Verify physician's orders for management of baby in incubator.

3. Explain procedure to mother/parents.
4. Prepare the incubator for placing the baby by cleaning it with soap & water & disinfecting.
5. Switch on the incubator & adjust the temperature at 36°C on Servo control mode* (By measuring skin temperature, the incubator heater turns on or off in order to keep skin temperature within preset range.)
6. Prewarm the incubator for 15 minutes as prewarming facilitates flow of warm air on body surface.
7. Undress the baby except for diapers for facilitating observation of baby through the clear plastic canopy.
8. Transfer baby to prepared incubator.
9. Check temperature of newborn & the incubator every hour until the temperature of baby is stabilized.
10. Record temperature, heart rate, respiration & oxygen saturation.
11. Change humidifier water every day.
12. Give care for baby by introducing hand through arm ports.
13. Permit mother/parents to see & bond with the baby according to hospital policy.
14. Weaning a baby is important & has to be taken care of. This is done by gradually decreasing the temperature of incubator & monitoring the infant's body according to hospital policy.
15. Do not tap incubator.

Care of Incubator

1. Humidity or Oxygen delivered to baby in an incubator is heated according to condition of baby.
2. Hoods of incubators are changed every 2 weeks (Place the date change & date when next change is due on plexiglass hood).
3. Incubators are checked & maintained by Bio-Medical Engineering every 6 months.
4. Wipe off all the spills with hospital approved disinfectant.
5. Clean inside & outside of incubator.
6. For inside area dampen a cloth with hospital approved disinfectant. Do not spray disinfectant with baby in incubator.

Factors Affecting Microenvironmental Temperature

1. **Room Temperature:** The effective environmental temperature inside a single walled incubator is estimated by subtracting 1°C from recorded incubator air temperature.
2. **Draughts:** Cold draughts from air conditioning vents should not strike directly on incubator wall nor should incubators be near cold windows.
3. **Sunlight:** Heat gain is possible from protracted exposure of incubator to sunlight from a window & serious elevation of body temperature may occur.
4. Relative Humidity.

CHAPTER 27

Care of Baby in Radiant Warmer

Introduction

Radiant warmer is the device used to maintain the temperature of the baby and to prevent hypothermia.

Prepare a bed at least 30 minutes before the baby arrives in the nursery to ensure the baby is received in a warm, Comfortable environment.

Steps of the Procedure

1. Clean the radiant warmer/incubator properly before use.
2. Switch on the main electrical supply.
3. Put the baby sheet on the bed. Arrange all necessary items near the bed.
4. Put the radiant warmer on the manual mode with 100% heater output so that the temperature of all items likely to come in contact with the baby, are warm.
5. Once the radiant warmer is ready. Switch to skin mode with desired setting.
6. Read temperature on display. Abdominal skin temperature should be 95.9° to 97.7° F (35.5° to 36.5°C).
7. Tape the probe onto the infant's abdomen b/w the umbilicus and xiphoid process in supine position and groin area in prone position.
8. Note the length of time of radiant waves.
9. Maintain the fluid and electrolyte balance with 30% extra fluid.
10. Place only one baby under each radiant warmer.
11. Check the temperature of the warmer and of the room every hour and adjust the temperature setting accordingly. Record the heater output in each shift (every 6 hours)
12. Move the baby with the mother as soon as the baby no longer requires frequent procedures and treatment.

For Disinfection

1. For daily cleaning of front panel use damp cloth soaked in mild detergent.
2. Do not use spirit or other chemicals.
3. Bassinet, cot should be disinfected daily using soap/detergent solution or disinfection solution.

CHAPTER 28

Total Parenteral Nutrition

Introduction

Parenteral nutrition is the intravenous administration of a solution of dextrose, amino acids, electrolytes, vitamins, insulin, thiamine, and trace elements in amounts that meet or exceed the patient's energy expenditure.

Purposes

To provide nutrition in concentrated form to the pediatric patient.

Indications

1. Large wounds
2. Short bowel syndrome
3. Enterocutaneous fistula
4. Inflammatory bowel disease
5. Ulcerative colitis
6. Mild-to-moderate hepatic failure

Patent access

- Central lines (including PICC lines) utilizing solution with final glucose concentration of 10% or higher.
- Peripheral lines (including midline catheters) utilizing solutions with final glucose concentration of 10% or lower.

Steps of the Procedure

1. Check the physician's written order in file.
2. Explain the procedure to the child/parents.
3. Check the blood chemistry value.
4. Handwashing.
5. Use the antiseptic technique while attaching the tubing.
6. Check the label on the solution with the patient's identification band. Positive patient identification is required prior to hanging the solution.
7. Connect new tubing and solution according to the access established.

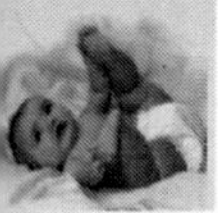

8. Established line using aseptic technique, connect the new tubing and solution to the already established line.
9. Establishing a new access using sterile techniques, a central line will be placed by the physician. Using aseptic techniques, a peripheral line will be initiated by nursing staff.
10. The rate is ordered by the physician. Connect the tubing to the Electronic regulator and adjust the rate accordingly.
11. Check to be certain that all connections are secure and that tubing and dressings are labeled with initials, date, and time.
12. During TPN infusion, nurses should observe to the patient's respiration, B/P temperature.
13. Check the blood glucose level as per doctor order.
14. No solution is to be hanged more than twenty-four (24) hours after the protective cap has been removed.
15. Change macrodrip tubing and connectors every 24 hours with the daily solution change.
16. Both central line and peripheral line site dressing changes will be done every 24-48 hours or as needed, if wet, and/or nonocclusive.
17. Use aseptic technique during dressing.
18. Weigh the patient daily with the same amount of clothing, using the same scale.
19. Maintain intake and output record.
20. Record parenteral nutrition fluid totals separate from other fluid intake.
21. Take and record vital signs as per the unit assessment standards.

CHAPTER 29

Gastric Lavage

Gastric lavage, also commonly called stomach pumping or gastric irrigation, is the process of cleaning out the contents of the stomach. A flexible tube is inserted through the nose, down the throat, and into the stomach and the contents of the stomach are suctioned out. The inside of the stomach is rinsed with a saline (salt water) solution.

Indications

1. Poisoning.
2. Specimen collection.
3. To relieve nausea and vomiting in case of acute dilation of stomach, pyloric stenosis and intestinal obstruction.
4. To clean the stomach as a preparation for surgery.

Equipments

- Infant feeding tube No. 6, 8, 9, Fr. According to the age of child.
- Mackintosh with towel/draw sheet.
- Syringe 5 cc.
- Stethoscope.
- Adhesive plaster.
- Normal saline/specific antidote as per order of the physician.
- Swab stick to clean the nostril.
- Kidney tray/paper bag.
- Clean gloves.
- Bowl with water.
- Specimen container.
- Empty bottle.
- Suction catheter and suction equipment in case of aspiration. I/V set for connection with empty bottle.

Steps of the Procedure

1. Check the written doctor order in file.
2. Explain the procedure to parents/child.
3. Provide the privacy.

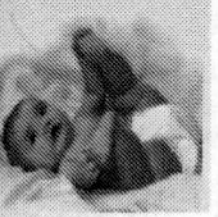

4. Assemble all the articles at bed side.
5. Perform handwashing.
6. Place mackintosh and towel below chin of the child.
7. Clean the nostrils with swab sticks.
8. Measure the tube placing from tip of the nose to earlobe and then up to Xiphoid process of the sternum.
9. Lubricate the tube with little lubricating jelly.
10. Insert the tube through the nostril of the child.
11. Emphasize need to mouth breath and swallow during the procedure.
12. Check the correct position of the tube in the stomach by injecting 3-4 cc air and ausculatate with stethoscope, placed over epigastric region.
13. Withdraw injecting air from the stomach and aspirate the gastric content.
14. Fix the tube with adhesive tape. When the tube is in, aspirate the gastric contents completely and save it for laboratory analysis. Label them properly and send it to the lab.
15. Normal saline are administered through Ryle's tube and via a siphoning action removed again.
16. In children, normal saline is used, as children are more at risk of developing hyponatremia if lavaged with water.
17. Collect the gastric specimen.
18. Remove the mackintosh and towel.
19. Clean the child's face with tissue paper.
20. Remove the gloves.
21. Waste materials dispose as per hospital policy.
22. Collect all the articles and clean. Keep in proper place.
23. Write in nursing notes, collect specimen in the sterile container, record specimen color, amount, date and time. Put your signature.

Tracheostomy Care

Definition

A tracheostomy is a surgical opening in the trachea the procedure may be done on an emergency basis or may be an elective one, and it may be combined with mechanical ventilation.

Three major factors must be considered in the care of the tracheostomy patient:

1. Humidification.
2. Mobilization of secretions.
3. Airway patency.

1. **Humidity:** The patient must be properly hydrated with oral or IV fluids to permit the mucosal surface to remain moist and to ensure that the viscid secretions remain atop the cilia. This will make the secretions thinner and more mobile. Instillation of sterile saline directly into the tracheostomy tube at intervals, usually before and during suctioning, may aid in loosening and keeping secretions moist.
2. **Mobilization of Secretions:** Many of the nursing skills employed are aimed at the mobilization of pulmonary secretions. Frequent turning, encouragement of deep breathing, and ambulation are important in the prevention of pulmonary complications. Regular chest physiotherapy and postural drainage are both very effective in the mobilization of secretions and should be used routinely during the postoperative period.
3. **Suctioning:** Suctioning is an uncomfortable procedure and is usually a frightening one for the patient. It is a procedure where both psychological and physiological defensive reflexes will come into play for the protection of the airway.

Articles Required

- Portable suction pump or tracheal wall suction.
- Disposable suction catheter, kits of appropriate size or single disposable suction catheters.
- Gloves.
- Basin.
- Small jar of sterile normal saline.

Steps of the Procedure

1. Gather your supplies and equipment.
2. Explain the procedure to patient/parents.
3. Wash your hands with surgical soap.

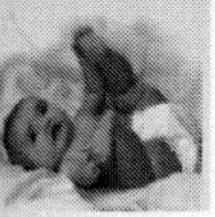

4. Pepare equipment, open kit or catheter pack, saline, etc.
5. Put on sterile gloves.
6. Remove sterile suction catheter from package.
7. Lubricate tip of catheter by dipping tip in sterile saline or by rolling in sterile water-soluble lubricant.
8. Be sure patient is preoxygenated.
9. Open suction port on swivel. If the patient is not on mechanical ventilation, disconnect from the supplemental oxygen source and humidifier.
10. If the patient is cooperative, ask him/her to take a deep breath and quickly but gently insert the catheter into the trachea. If resistance is felt, withdraw the catheter slightly. The catheter control valve is left open or not depressed during insertion so that no suction is applied during insertion.
11. Apply intermittent suction. Rotate the catheter between your thumb and forefinger during withdrawal.
12. As soon as the catheter is withdrawn, reconnect to the ventilator, or oxygen supply source. Reoxygenate the patient.
13. Clear the catheter with saline.
14. Repeat procedure if necessary until airway is clear of secretions.

Record and Report

- Quantity, color, and consistency of secretions.
- Number of times the patient required suctioning per shift.
- Patient's tolerance.
- Condition of skin around the tracheostomy site.
- Any complications associated with the suctioning procedure.
- The volume of air required to obtain a cuff seal.

CHANGING TRACHEOSTOMY DRESSINGS

It is very important to change tracheostomy dressings as soon as they get soiled.

While changing the tracheostomy ties or holders, one nurse holds the tube in place while the other removes the old ties or holder and replaces them with new.

Articles Required

- Tracheostomy dressings.
- Clean tracheostomy ties with ½ -strength hydrogen peroxide/normal saline.
- Dry sterile pad or towel.
- **NOTE:** Plain sterile gauze pads should not be used to create tracheostomy dressings, as fibers that become loose may be aspirated into the airway.

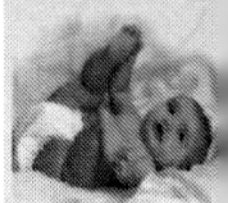

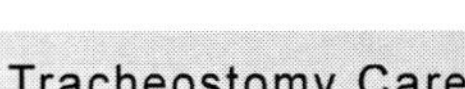

Steps of the Procedure

1. Remove old dressing, being careful to keep tracheostomy tube in place.
2. Clean around tube at stoma site with hydrogen peroxide/saline solution.
3. Place clean tracheostomy dressing under the flange, inserted from below.
4. Change dressing as necessary.

CARE OF SKIN AROUND TRACHEOSTOMY

Care of the skin around the stoma site should be considered one of the more important procedures in the care of the tracheostomy patient. The new surgical site needs to be cleaned and dressed frequently as it heals. As the incision heals the frequency will decrease.

Articles Required

1. Cotton-tipped swabs.
2. Normal saline or ½ –strength hydrogen peroxide.

Steps of the Procedure

1. Gather all necessary supplies.
2. Wash your hands with surgical soap and water.
3. Inspect the site around the tracheostomy stoma for signs of skin breakdown, infection, or irritation.
4. Moisten the swabs in either the peroxide solution or with normal saline.
5. With a rolling motion, clean the skin area around the stoma and under the flange of the tube.
6. Pat dry with a clean dry swab or pad.
7. Replace tracheostomy dressing.

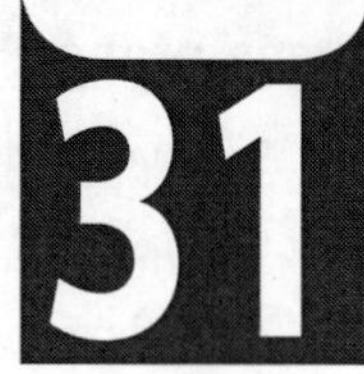

Chest Tube Insertion

Definition

It is the procedure of inserting chest tubes into the thoracic cavity and enclosing a close drainage system to re-expand the involved lung and to remove excess air, fluid and blood.

Purpose

1. To restore the negative intrathoracic pressure needed for lung re-expansion following surgery or trauma.
2. To treat pneumothorax and hemothorax.

General Instruction

1. This procedure is performed by a doctor and assisted by a registered nurse.
2. Strict aseptic technique has to be followed during the procedure.
3. Emergency resuscitation equipment should be in reach.
4. Tubes should be clamped during insertion.
5. Long tubes should be anchored to the bed.
6. All connections are to be sealed.
7. The level of the drainage bag should be kept lower than the chest.

Equipment

- Trolley containing.
  - Chest seal drainage system
- A tray with
  - Chest drainage tube
  - Scalpel blade
  - Silk suture
  - Suture set with sterile scissors
- An injection tray with:
  - 10 ml syringe
  - 5 ml syringe
  - Needles

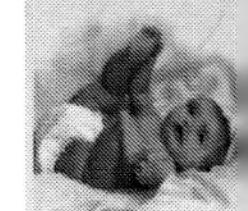

- Local anesthetic (xylocaine 2%)

- Other articles
  - Betadine
  - Leukoplast
  - Sterile gloves
  - Scissors
  - Specimen tubes

Steps of the Procedures

1. Explain procedure to the child/family.
2. Record vital signs.
3. Wash and dry hands according to surgical asepsis.
4. Add sterile water to the drainage system uptill the specified level.
5. Ensure that the chest tube is 2 cm below the water level in the bottle/bag.
6. Ensure that the cork is tightly fixed.
7. Clamp tubing until equipment is connected.
8. Ensure that the tubing is long enough to allow free movement.
9. Place the child in fowlers or semi fowlers position.
10. Observe and the child throughout procedure.
11. Open sterile equipment and assist the physician in inserting the chest tube.
12. If pus is present collect the specimen in sterile specimen bottle.
13. Apply dry dressing to cannula insertion site.
14. Throughout entire procedure, monitor child vital signs and signs of distress.
15. Ensure that child is left feeling comfortable and rearrange clothing's and bedding.
16. Document procedure in nurse's records.

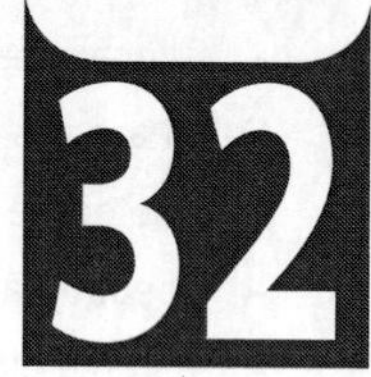

Electrocardiogram (ECG)

Introduction

An electrocardiogram is a graphic record of the electrical impulses that are generated by external surface of the body where they are detected by electrodes and measured by galvanometer.

The SA node (pacemaker of the heart) initiates each heart beat by discharging an electrical impulse. As this electrical impulse spreads over the atria and ventricles, the atria contracts and is followed by ventricles contraction (depolarization). As the wave of contraction passes off, atria and ventricles relax (repolarization). This process normally takes place with each heart beat (80-120 times per minute).

Articles Required

- Electrodes
- Gel
- Gauge
- ECG Machine.

Steps of the Procedures

1. No special preparation of the child is necessary for taking ECG.
2. If the patient is ignorant of the procedure, the nurse should explain the procedure to the child and reassure him that the procedure is absolutely safe.
3. In intensive care units, the cardiac rhythm is monitored continuously by a cardiac monitor in order to detect ECG changes that may indicate myocardial ischemia.
4. There must be good contact between the child skin and the electrodes. This can be assured by applying electrodes jelly to the skin where the electrode is attached.
5. The child should wear no ornaments on the body during ECG. If it is unavoidable, care should be taken that the leads should not come in contact with the ornaments.
6. The child position is also important and can affect tracings. He should lie flat and as relaxed as possible, because any movement or muscular twitching recorded by the machine may alter the tracings.
7. Before each ECG, the machine should be checked for proper standardization. When the standardization button is pressed, there should be a defection of 10 mm on the graph. This means a spike made will be of two large squares.
8. It is important that machine should be properly grounded to prevent interference with the recording.

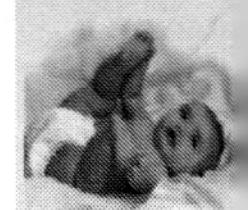

9. There are specific position for the placement of the chest leads and the nurses should know where they are. The improper placement of the chest leads can greatly distort the tracing and alter the diagnosis.
   a. V1 – In the fourth intercostal space to the right of the sternum.
   b. V2 – In the fourth intercostal space to the left of the sternum.
   c. V3 – Midway between V2 and V4.
   d. V4 – In the fifth intercostal space in the midclavicular line on the left side.
   e. V5 – In the same horizontal position as V4 in the anterior auxiliary line. On the left side.
   f. V6 – In the same horizontal position as V4 in the auxiliary line, on the left side.
10. No other electric equipment should work in the monitoring area.

CHAPTER 33

Blood Transfusion Therapy

Introduction

Blood transfusions are therapeutic measures used to restore blood or plasma volume after extensive hemorrhage, or trauma; to increase the number and concentration of red blood cells in persons with anemia in order to increase the oxygen carrying capacity of their blood; and to treat shock.

Indication

1. Acute blood loss of more than 20- 30%.
2. Severe anemia.
3. Septic shock.
4. Pre or postoperatively.
5. To provide platelets, plasma or clotting factors.
6. To provide nutritional elements in blood.
7. To reduce toxicity and to increase resistance.

Equipment

A tray containing.

- Blood transfusion set.
- Normal saline.
- Syringe – 5 ml and 10 ml.
- Guaze pieces.
- Three way.
- Kidney tray.
- Sterile gloves.
- TPR tray.
- Blood unit to be transfused.
- I/V Stand.

General Guidelines

- Record vital signs before administering blood to establish base line data for post transfusion comparison, then every 15 minutes for 1 hour while blood is being transfused.
- Cross checking the reaction forms and blood packs before transfusing the blood.
- Administer the first 50 ml of blood slowly.
- Administer blood through an appropriate filter to eliminate particle in the blood and prevent the precipitation of the formed elements, gently shake the blood bag frequently.
- Infuse a unit of blood within four hours.
- If a reaction of any type is suspected, take vital signs, stop the transfusion maintain a patent line with normal saline and new tubings, notify the physician.

Steps of the Procedures

1. Explain the procedure to the parents/child.
2. Verify that informed consent has been obtained.
3. Offer bedpan or urinal if required.
4. Verify the physician order, noting the indication, rate of infusion and any premedication.
5. Assemble the articles near the patient's bed.
6. Spread the mackintosh and draw sheet under the area of the child where cannula is inserted.
7. Compare the blood bag and patient's treatment chart or patient's identification tag for preventing the incompatibility.
8. Take base line vital signs.
9. Do thorough hand washing.
10. Open the blood bag without contamination of the tip.
11. The blood should be at room temperature.
12. Connect the tubing to the bag after removing the seal and flush the line completely to prevent air entry.
13. Flush the cannula with saline and ensure its patency.
14. Using aseptic technique, attach the distal set to the IV catheter or cannula.
15. Adjust the drip rate, as prescribed.
16. Remain with the patient during the first 5 min and then obtain vital signs.
17. Obtain vital signs in 15 minutes then again in 30 minutes, and then hourly while the transfusion is being infused or as prescribed.
18. A mid transfusion diuretic is to be given, if prescribed.
19. After transfusing the whole blood, stop the flow.
20. Record vital sign of the patient.

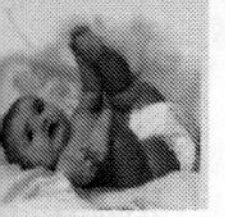

Action at Transfusion Reaction

- Stop the transfusion immediately if signs or symptoms of a transfusion reaction occur.
- Do not flush the tubing with normal saline solution.
- Disconnect the administration set from the IV catheter.
- Obtain vital signs and auscultate heart and breath sounds.
- Notify physician as soon as the blood has been stopped and patient has been assessed.

After Care

- Discard the empty blood container and administration set in the proper receptacle according to the hospital policy.
- Document all vital signs, response and interventions completely.
- Continue monitoring patient for 30 minutes.

Complications

Immediate reactions

- Hemolytic reactions.
- Febrile reactions.
- Allergic reactions.
- Circulatory overload.
- Air emboli.
- Hypothermia.

Delayed reaction

- Transmission of infection.
- Delayed hemolytic reactions.

CHAPTER 34

Lumbar Puncture

Introduction

The cerebrospinal fluid is formed through the chorio villi, in each of the four ventricles of the brain and it circulates freely through the ventricles, the subarachnoid space and the central canal of the spinal cord. It is then absorbed into the venous circulation via superior sagittal sinus.

During development the vertebral column outgrows the spinal cord. In adult, the spinal cord ends at the lower border of the first lumbar vertebra; but in the newborn infant it ends slightly at the lower level at the level of the third lumbar vertebra. The dural and arachnoid sacs extend up to the level of the second sacral vertebra and this cavity contains the CSF. Thus the region between the second lumbar vertebra and the second sacral vertebra is suitable for the withdrawal of CSF, as there is no danger of injury to the spinal cord.

Definition

A lumbar puncture is the insertion of a needle into the lumbar region of the spine, in such a manner that the needle enters the lumbar arachnoid space of the spinal canal below the level of the spinal cord, so that the cerebrospinal fluid can be withdrawn or a substance can be therapeutically or diagnostically injected.

Purpose of Lumbar Puncture

- To administer spinal anesthesia before surgery in the lower half of the body.
- To administer medication into the spinal cord as in the case of meningitis.
- To remove fluid (CSF, blood pus, etc.) contained in the subarachnoid space, thereby reducing the intracranial pressure.
- To remove a sample of CSF for laboratory examinations in order to diagnose disease.
- To measure the pressure of CSF and to determine whether the lumbar sub arachnoid space is in communication with the ventricles of brain.
- To remove CSF and to replace it with air, oxygen or radio opaque substances for diagnostic X-rays in order to locate tumors or other brain disorders.

Complications

- Injury to the spinal cord and spinal nerves.
- Infection introduced into the spinal cavity which may give rise to meningitis.
- Leakage of CSF through the puncture site and lowering the intracranial pressure and may cause post puncture headaches.

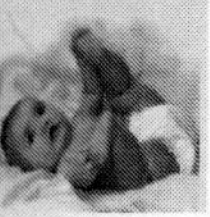

- Damage to the intervertebral disks.
- Local pain, edema and hematoma at the puncture site.
- Temperature elevation.
- Rapid reduction in the intracranial space.

Site of the Lumbar Puncture and the Positioning of the Patient

In lumbar puncture a needle is inserted into the lumbar area (L3-4) is the preferred site of the subarachnoid space. The patient is placed in a side lying position at the edge of the table or bed. The patient's body should be in the fetal attitude (C shaped) with full flexion of the spine. In the neonate, the sitting position may be preferable. To restrain an older infant or young child in the lateral recumbent position, the nurse may place one hand behind the child's neck or one arm around the neck and grasp the legs, while placing the other arm around the buttocks and grasping the hands.

Preparation of Articles

A sterile tray containing:

- LP needles – 2 sizes with their stilette.
- Sponge holding forceps.
- Syringe (5 ml) with needles to give anesthesia.
- Small bowl to take cleaning lotion.
- Specimen bottle.
- Cotton balls, gauze pieces and cotton pads.
- Gloves, gown and masks.
- Dressing towels or slit towel.
- Three way adapter, manometer and tubing to measure the pressure of the CSF if required.

An unsterile tray containing

- Mackintosh and towel.
- Kidney tray and paper bag.
- Spirit, iodine, tr. Benzoin, etc.
- Lignocaine 2 percent.
- Sterile normal saline to fill in the manometer.
- Adhesive plaster and scissors.

General Instructions

1. Strict aseptic techniques are to be followed.
2. Child should be placed in a position that will widen the interverteberal space.
3. Uncooperative patients and children are to be restrained during the procedure.
4. The patient should be placed near the edge of the bed.

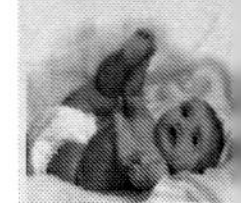

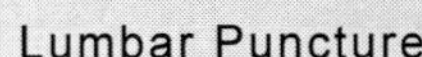

5. The LP needles should be sharp, small in size and not curved.
6. After the lumbar puncture, the patient should lie flat on the bed.
7. The CSF collected should be sent to the laboratory without any delay.
8. Drugs to be injected must be warmed to body temperature and it should be injected very slowly.
9. Local anesthesia may be given subcutaneously at the injection site prior to the procedure or a patch impregnated with lidocaine is applied to the skin 3 hours before the procedure.

Preparation of the Patient

- Explain the procedure to the parents.
- Monitor vitals before the procedure.
- Prepare the skin as for a surgical procedure. Skin is disinfected with spirit and iodine just before doing the spinal puncture.
- Put on clean and loose garments.
- Arrange the articles at the bedside table.
- Fold back the upper garments above the waist line and the lower garments below the hip.
- Protect the bed with mackintosh.

After Care of the Procedure

- As soon as the needle is withdrawn, seal the puncture site to prevent leakage of CSF.
- Place the child comfortable on the bed in a supine position for 12 to 24 hours.
- If the patient develops post puncture headache, the following precautions are taken.
- Darken the room.
- Give plenty of oral fluids.
- Administer analgesics.
- Raise the foot end of the bed.
- Watch for patient's color, pulse, respiration, blood pressure and other signs of complications.
- Record the procedure on the patient's chart with date and time.
- The specimens of CSF collected should be sent to the laboratory without any delay with proper labels and requisition form.
- If there are no complications observed, the patient may be allowed to be upright after 8 to 12 hours.

Neonatal Advanced Life Support

Introduction

A child who is struggling to breath but conscious should be transported immediately to an advanced life support (ALS) facility.

The child maintaining whatever position affords the most comfort. However, attempting to transport a child by automobile wastes valuable time in obtaining help, transport by and emergency medical service (EMS) is recommended or preferred.

Services in larger communities can institute ALS immediately or enroute to a medical facility.

Ask following questions within few seconds of birth.

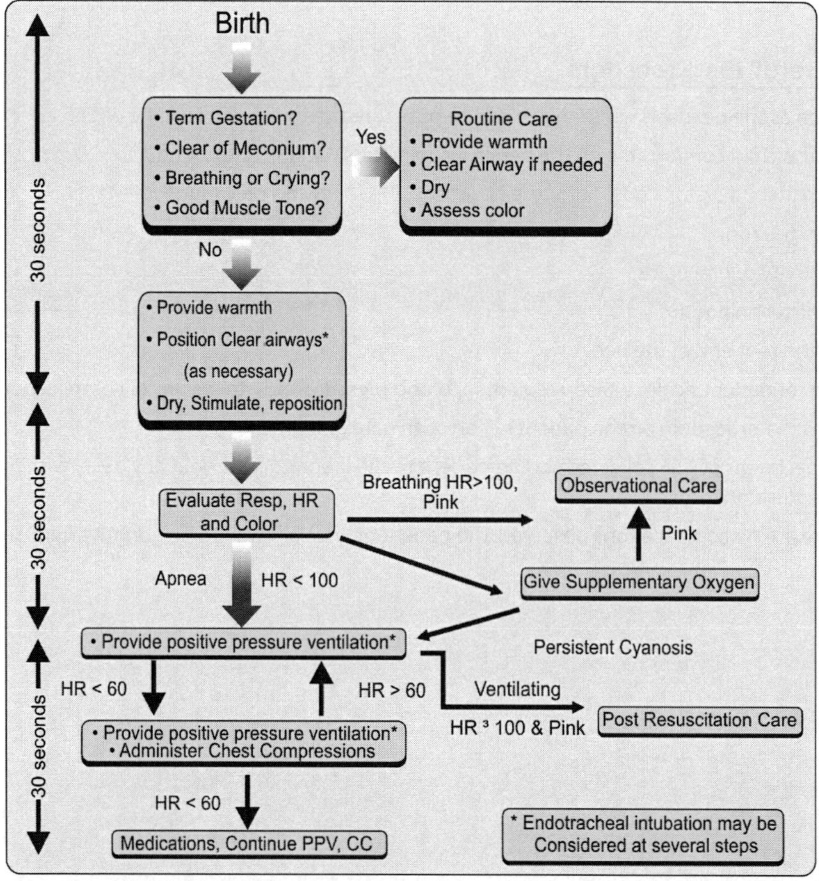

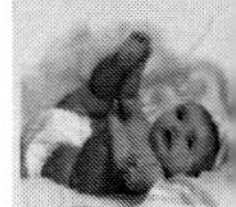

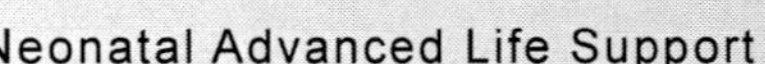

- Is the baby born at Term gestation?
- Is the amniotic fluid clear of Meconium?
- Is the baby breathing or Crying?
- Is the Muscle tone good?

Initial Steps

- Provide warmth.
- Position: clear airway as necessary.
- Dry, stimulate and reposition.

Provide Warmth

- Place under radiant warmer.
- Leave the baby uncovered under warmer
  - To allow full visualization
  - To permit radiant heat to reach the baby

Premature babies more vulnerable to cold stress because of

- Larger body surface area, thin skin.
- Less subcutaneous fat, decreased metabolic response.
- Monitor for hyperthermia.

Position clear airway as necessary

- Sniffing position.
- Use a shoulder roll.

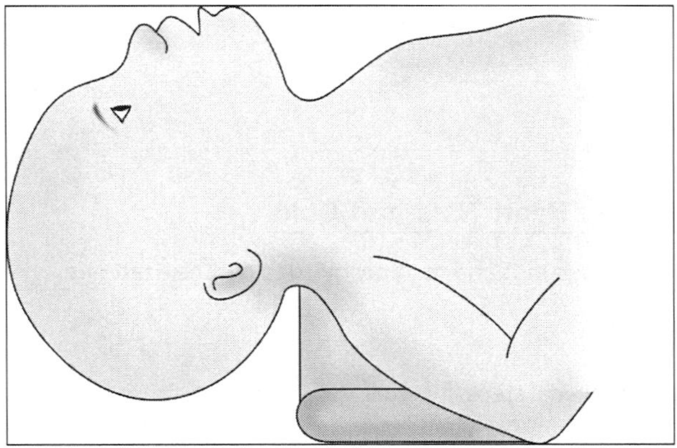

Clear Airway

- Secretions can be removed from airway with a towel/bulb syringe/suction catheter.
- In presence of copious secretions, turn face to side.

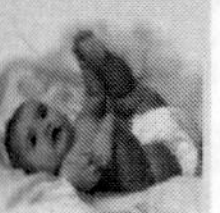

- Apply gentle suction with pressure < 100 mm Hg.
- Always do suction of mouth before nose (M before N).
- Stimulation of posterior pharynx cause vagal stimulation and bradycardia. If bradycardia occurs, stop suction.

Dry, Stimulate and Reposition

- Use pre-warmed absorbent towels or blankets.
- Keep head in 'sniffing' position to maintain good airway.
- Suction and drying will provide sufficient stimulation.
- If inadequate respiration, then additional tactile stimulation given briefly by.
- Slapping or flicking the soles of the feet.
- Gently rubbing the back, trunk or extremities.

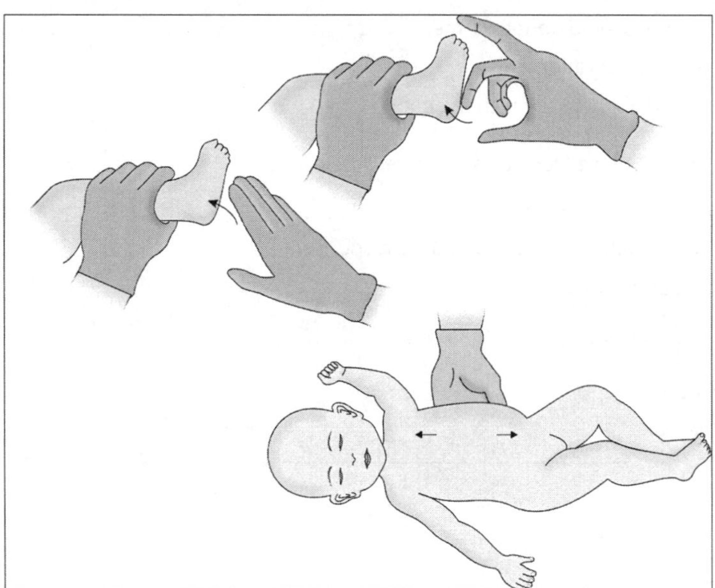

Evaluate: Respiration, Heart Rate and Color

Count the heart beats for 6 seconds and multiply by 10 to get the heart rate.

Give oxygen, as necessary

Give free flow oxygen after initial steps if.

- Baby is breathing well.
- Heart rate > 100 bpm.
- Central cyanosis.

Oxygen can be given by

- Oxygen tubing with cupped hand.

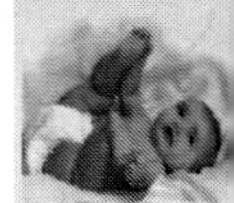

- Oxygen mask.
- Flow-inflating bag and mask.
- T – piece resuscitator.

  Gradually withdraw oxygen when baby turns pink.

Further evaluation

- Respiration.
- Heart Rate.

  Count for 6 seconds and multiply by 10.

Feel pulse at base of umbilicus or auscultate

≥ 100 bpm-normal.

- Color.

If baby is not improving, then go for positive pressure ventilation according to the flow chart.

1. Appropriate size mask.
2. Appropriate size ET tube.
3. ET suction catheter.
4. Wall suction.
5. Shoulder roll.
6. Adhesive/dynaplast cut in the shape of 'E' or 'H'.
7. Cardiac monitor or at least a pulse oxymeter.
8. Neonatal stethoscope.

S. No.	Weight of the neonate (GM)	Gestational age (weeks)	Internal diameter of the ET tube (MM)	Size of the suction catheter
1.	Below 1000	Below 28	2.5	5 or 6
2.	1000 – 2000	28 – 34	3	6 or 8
3.	2000 – 3000	34 – 38	3.5	8
4.	Above 3000	Above 38	3.5 – 4	8 or 10

Points to Remember for ET Intubations

- Pre oxygenate before intubation PPV with 100% oxygen.
- Deliver free flow oxygen during intubation.
- Not more than 20 sec per attempt : not more than 3 attempts.
- Ventilate with Bag and mask with 100% oxygen in between attempts.

Insertion of ET Tube

- Insert ET tube holding in the right hand.

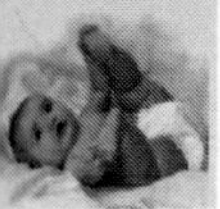

Bag and Mask Ventilation in the Newborn

Indications for bag mask (positive pressure) ventilation

a. Apnea.

b. Heart rate less than 100 bpm.

c. Signs of respiratory distress:
   - Increased work of breathing/chest retraction.
   - Nasal flaring.
   - Tachypnea.
   - Grunting.
   - Central Cyanosis.

Chest compression should be started if heart rate is less than 60 bpm despite 30 sec of effective positive- pressure ventilation. Endotracheal intubation at this time may help to ensure adequate ventilation and facilitate the coordination of ventilation and chest compressions.

Endotracheal Intubation

Indications

- Prolonged PPV required.
- Bag and mask ineffective: inadequate chest expansion.
- If chest compressions required: intubation may facilitate coordination and efficiency of ventilation.
- Tracheal suction required: for example, MSAF.
- Diaphragmatic hernia.
- Use of drugs through ET tube.

Articles Required

- Self inflating bag attached to 100% source gas.

Introduce through the Right Angle of the Mouth

- Keep glottis in view.
- Insert when vocal cords are apart.
- Do not push through vocal cords.
- If cords are together wait, if do not open within 20 sec stop and ventilate with bag and mask.

Chest Compression

Also referred to as external cardiac massage.

Rhythmic compressions of sternum that

- Compress the heart against the spine.

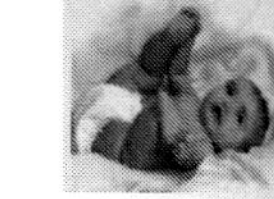

- Increase the intrathoracic pressure.
- Circulate blood to the vital organs.

Indication

Heart rate less then 60 bpm despite 30 sec of effective positive-pressure ventilation.

Why chest compression

- Myocardium is depressed because of poor oxygen levels-low cardiac output.
- Mechanical pumping of heart required to improve perfusion to the lungs.

Requirements

1. Chest compressions and PPV should be simultaneous.
2. Two people.

Techniques

(a) Thumb technique (Preferred).

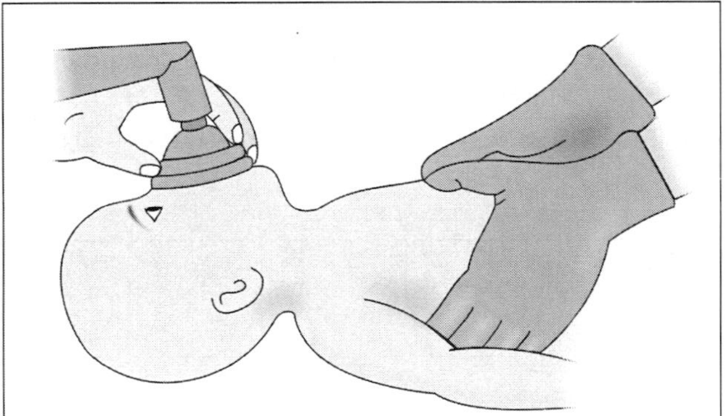

(b) Two finger technique

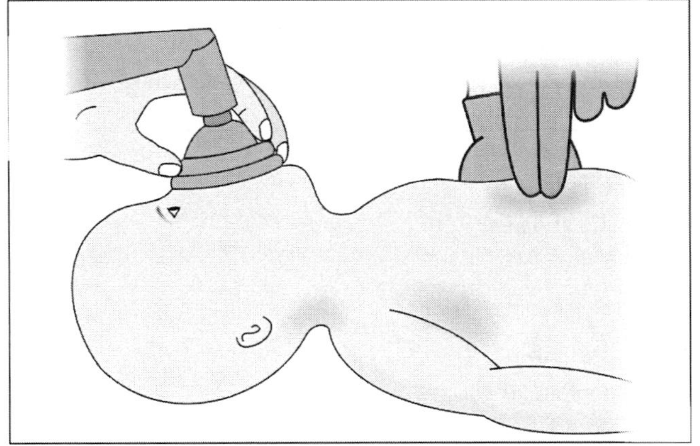

Position of thumb or fingers on the chest

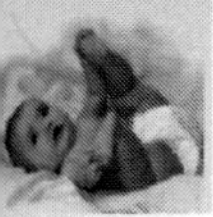

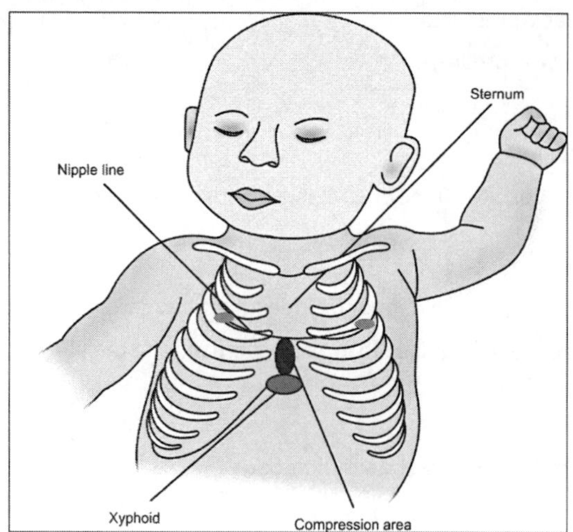

Position of fingers

- 1 cm below the nipple line.
- Feel the xyphoid process, and place fingers just above it.
- The rhythm for co-ordination between two resuscitations (one doing chest compression and other doing bag mask ventilation) is given below:

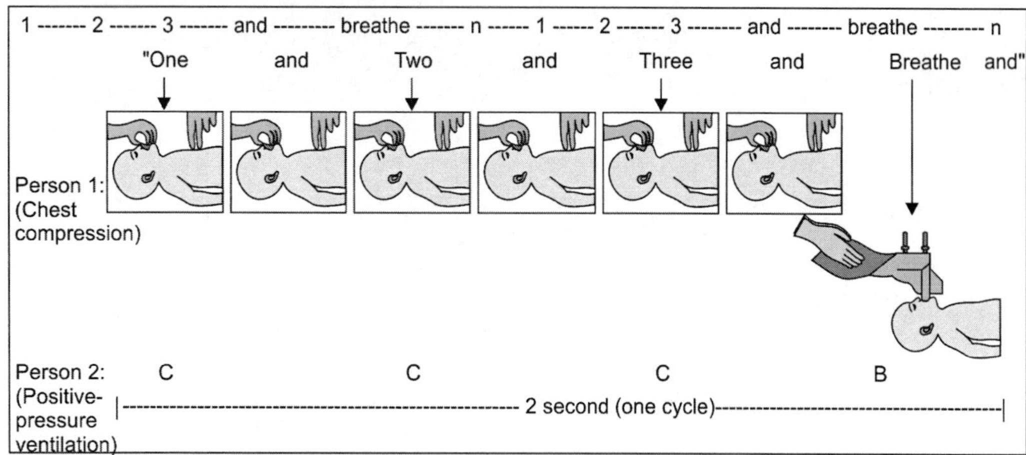

When to stop chest compressions

- After approx. 30 sec of CC and PPV
  - Count heart rate.
  - If > 60 bpm stop chest compressions.
- Continue PPV at 40-60 bpm till
  - Baby breathing spontaneously.
  - Heart rate > 100 and.
  - Baby pink.

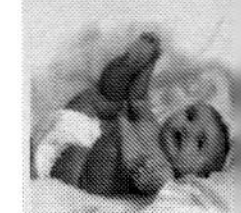

Medications

Indications for medications: despite administration of effective chest compression and effective positive – pressure ventilation with 100% oxygen.

- Heart rate is below 60 bpm.

Epinephrine

- Cardiac stimulant
  - Increases strength and rate of cardiac contractions.
  - Causes peripheral vasoconstriction.
  - It is indicated when HR remains < 60 bpm after 30 sec of effective PPV and another 30 sec of coordinated chest compression and ventilation.
- Available concentration 1:1000.
- Dilute it 10 times to make it 1:10.000.
- 1 ml of 1:10000 with 9 ml of water for injections.
- Dose : 0.1 – 0.3 ml/kg of 1:10,000.
- Preferred route : Intravenously while IV access is being obtained may give endotracheally: dose : 0.3 – 1.0 ml/kg of 1:10, 000 solutions.

After 30 seconds of administration and continued PPV and CC

- HR should increase to > 60 bpm, if no response repeat the dose every 3-5 minutes.

CHAPTER 36

Care of Baby on Ventilator

Introduction

The first several days after birth particularly first 72 hours after birth are critical for survival. Babies needing ventilator support require diligent medical and nursing care. The nurse-to-baby ratio for a critically ventilated neonate should ideally 1:1 and definitely not less than 1:2.

Definition: Normal respiration begins with the contraction of diaphragm and respiratory muscles to create negative pressure in the chest. A vacuum is created and the air flows in, when a ventilator is used positive pressure forces air into the lungs. The positive forces are necessary for the gas exchange and to keep alveoli open.

Purpose: To establish and maintain effective ventilation.

- To prevent complication associated with artificial ventilation.
- To ensure position and patency of endotracheal tube/ tracheostomy tube.
- To clear and remove secretions from airway.

General Instructions

- Nurses caring for patient on ventilator should have basic knowledge of pulmonary physiology.
- Nurses should have complete understanding of ventilator functions, awareness about potential complications and intervention to be taken in emergencies.
- Patient on continuous mechanical ventilation should never be left unattended.
- Vital signs should be checked & recorded hourly or as required.
- Suctioning should be performed under aseptic technique.
- Sterile catheter and gloves should be used for performing suctioning every time.
- Size of catheter should be less than half the diameter of endotracheal /trachostomy tube.
- Suction tubing should be kept transparent so that nature of aspirate can be observed.
- Ensure that vacuum pressure is not more than 100 mmhg in children.
- Nurse should provide gentle oral mucosa care daily to prevent pressure ulcers on baby,s lip or tongue.
- Inflation of endotracheal/tracheostomy tube to be monitored regularly.
- Functioning of ventilator alarms must be checked at beginning of each shift. Ventilator setting to be checked & recorded every hour.
- Tubing's leading from ventilator to patient must be checked at least every hour and Accumulated moisture to be removed.
- Humidifier to be kept adequately filled with sterile distilled water.
- In presence of possible ventilator fault nurse must always first check clinical state of patient. If this is satisfactory then proceed to detect fault.

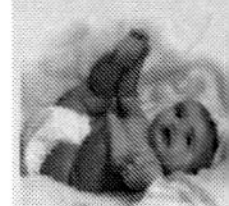

- If patient shows signs of insufficient ventilation the nurse must start manual ventilation whilst waiting for assistance.

Preparation of Articles

1. Ventilator tubing- inspiratory limb(2), Expiratory limb(2)
2. Water traps(2)
3. Y-connections
4. Healing wire
5. Flow sensor
6. Hundifier
7. Mouth Piere
8. Temperature wire/Probe
9. Ventilator
10. Sterile Sheets
11. Gown, Gloves, Mask
12. Power Supply
13. Intubation Tray

Types of Mechanical Ventilators

Mechanical ventilators can be:

1. **Negative Pressure Mechanical Ventilator:** Negative pressure ventilator exert a negative pressure on the external chest. Decreasing the intratnoracic pressure during inspiration allows air flow into the lungs, filling to its volume. Most common type of negative pressure ventilator is iron lung but they are not used now days.
2. **Positive Pressure Ventilators:** Positive Pressure ventilators inflate the lungs by exerting positive pressure in the airway, forcing the alveoli to expand during inspiration. Expiration occurs passively.

Three types of Positive Pressure Ventilators

A. **Pressure cycled ventilation:** They deliver the volume of gas to the airway using positive pressure during inspiration until a present pressure is reached.

B. **Volume cycled ventilator:** They deliver a preset tidal volume of inspired gas. The tidal Volume that has been preseuted is delivered to client regardless of the pressure required to deliver this volume.

C. **Time-Cycled Ventilators:** They terminate when time has elapsed.

D. **Flow Cycled Ventilators:** They are tiggled to stop when a present flow rate has been achieved.

Modes

1. Controlled Mechanical Ventilation (CMV)

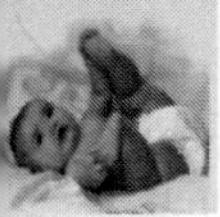

2. Assist-control ventilation (A/c)
3. Synchronized intermittent Mandatory (SIMU)
4. Pressure support ventilation (PSV)

1. **Controlled Mechanical Ventilation (CMV):** In this mode, the ventilator provides a mechanical breath on a present timing. Patient's respiratory efforts is ignored. This is generally uncomfortable for children and adults who are conscious and is usually only used in an unconscious patient.
2. **Assist Controlled Ventilation (ACV):** In this mode, the ventilator provides a mechanical breath with either a present tidal volume or peak pressure every time the patients initates a breath. However the initiation timing is the same both provide a ventilator breath with every patient effort. In most ventilators, a backup minimum breath rate can be in the event that patient becomes apnoeic. An alarm can be set if the ventilator cycles too frequently.
3. **Synchronized Intermittent Mandatory Volume (SIMV):** In this mode, the ventilator provides a pre set mechanical breath (Pressure or Volume limited) every specified number of seconds (determined by dividing the respiratory rate of 12 results in a 5-second cycled time). Within that cycle time the ventilator waits for the patient to initiate a breath using either a pressure or a flow sensor. When the ventilator sense the first patient breathing attempt within the cycle. It delivers a preset ventilator breath. If the patient fails to initiate a breath the ventilator delivers a mechanical breath at the end of a breath cycle. However SIMV breath within a breath the ventilator deliver a mechanical breath at the end of a breath cycle. However SIMV do not trigger another SIMV breath within a breath cycle if there are additional spontaneous breaths.
4. **Pressure Support Ventilation (PSV):** When a patient attempts to breath spontaneously through an endotracheal tube, the narrowed diameter of the airway results in a higher airflow resistance, thus a higher work of breathing PSV is a method to decrease the work of breathing in between the ventilator mandated breaths by providing an elevated pressure by spontaneous breathing that "supports" ventilation during inspiration. SIMV might be combined with PSV so that additions breaths beyond the SIMV programmed breaths are supported.

Procedure

1. **Care of ETT/Tracheostomy Tube:** Secure positioning of ETT/tracheostomy tube with adhesive plaster. Inflate cuff once correct positioning has been confirmed. Cuff is inflated with air using a syringe until a 'hiss' is heard on auscultation.
2. **Maintaining ventilation:** Effects of ventilation are assessed by observing patient color, chest movement, BP, pulse rate, oxygen saturation. Ventilator make characteristic sounds during inspiration & expiration which nurse must be capable of identifying. Ensure patient has adequate fluid & calorie intake. Administer sedation as prescribed to ensure adequate artificial ventilation & promotion of rest.
3. **Signs of adequate ventilation:** Improvement in skin color, oxygen saturation more than 90% and rhythmic expansion of chest with expiratory phase longer than inspiratory phase indicates adequate ventilation. Change in pulse rate may indicate decreased cardiac output due to increased intra thoracic pressure. A drop in blood pressure may reflect decreased cardiac output.

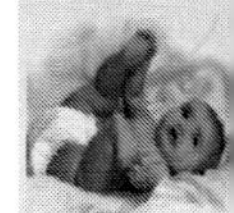

4. **Signs of inadequate ventilation:** Breathing occurs out of sequence with ventilation & pt is restless, diaphoretic, flushed or cyanosed. First signs of ventilatory inadequacy & hypoxia may be tachycardia & hypertension. If change in recording of ventilatory volume occurs check airway pressure & rate of ventilation. If increase in minute volume, check the leaks in cuffs seal, connection&tubing's.

   If decrease in minute volume, check for leaks in circuit. If increase in peak airway pressure occur check for obstruction such as secretions, kinking, pooling of water, pneumothorax.

5. **Suctioning:** Explain procedure to pt/family Frequency of suction to be carried out depending on pt's pulmonary state. Tracheal suction is an aseptic procedure.

   Sterile catheter & one sterile glove to be used for each suctioning session. Suction is applied while catheter is being withdrawn using intermittent technique not more than 10 to 15 seconds. When secretions are tenacious, instil 1 to 3 ml.sterile normal saline 0.9 % into endotracheal/tracheostomy tube to liquefy & make removal easier.

6. **Weaning:** Inform patient that this is a progressive step in treatment. Repeatedly encourage & reassure patient to avoid fear. Withhold sedation & muscle relaxant as ordered by doctor. Watch for respiratory distress, hypoxia, tachycardia, tachypnea, cyanosis, and hypotension& drop in o2 saturation.

7. **Routine nursing care:**

   (a) Give daily bed bath & change bed linen, if soiled.

   (b) Provide 2 hourly attentions to pressure sites by turning & repositioning of patient.

   (c) Provide 4 hourly oral hygiene & whenever needed.

   (d) Provide 4 hourly eye care.

   (e) Check & record vital signs every hour.

   (f) Measure I/V infusions & fluid intake every hour.

   (g) Measure blood loss, urine, nasogastric, aspirate etc every hour.

   (h) Change drainage bags, chest drainage bottles & tubing's as required.

   (i) Maintain intake /output chart for every shift

   (j) Assess bowel action every third day 8 hourly wound dressing should be done.

   (k) Change I/V administration sets & dressing of puncture sites every day.

   (l) Change suction bottle & connecting tubing every day.

   (m) Record pt's condition & events that have occurred during each shift in nurse progress sheet.

   (n) Give detailed hand over to nurse on following shift.

8. **Psychological aspect of patient care:** Endeavour to allay patient & relative's anxiety, fears & clear doubts as necessary. Motivate pt & relatives to participate in daily care activities. Promote good relationship with patient's family & encourage them to express fears, stress factor & feeling.

CHAPTER 37

Drug Dose Calculations

Clark's Rule: Clark's rule uses weight in pounds never in kilograms.

$$\text{Child Dose} = \frac{\text{Adult Dose} \times \text{Weight}}{150}$$

Example: 11 Yr. old girl weighing 70 Lbs, Adult Dose of Althrocin is 500 mg.

$$\text{So Child Dose} = \frac{500 \times 70}{150}$$

$$= 235 \text{ mg}$$

Young's Rule: Young's rule uses age (to remember easily, the word young refers to age)

$$\text{Child Dose} = \frac{\text{Adult Dose} \times \text{Age}}{\text{Age} + 12}$$

$$\text{Drug to be administered} = \frac{\text{What we want} \times \text{Amount Dissolved}}{\text{What we have}}$$

Example: 11 Yr. old girl weighing 70 Lbs, Adult Dose of Althrocin is 500 mg.

$$\text{So Child Dose} = \frac{500 \times 11}{11 + 12}$$

$$= 240 \text{ mg}$$

Example: Calculate dose of amoxicillin suspension in mls for otitis media for a 1 yr old child weighing 22 lb. The dose required is 40 mg/kg/day divided BD and suspension available in concentration of 400mg/5ml.

Solution: *Step 1:* Convert pounds to kg

$$= \frac{22\text{1b} \times 1\text{kg}}{2.2\text{1b}}$$

$$= 10 \text{ Kg}$$

Step 2: Calculate dose required by Child

10 Kg x 40 mg/kg/day

= 400 mg/day

Step 3: Divide the dose by frequency

$$= \frac{400 \text{ mg/day}}{2(\text{BD})}$$

$$= 200 \text{ mg/dose}$$

Step 4: Convert the dose into ml.

$$= \frac{200 \text{ mg/dose}}{400 \text{ mg/day} \times 5 \text{ ml}}$$

$$= 2.5 \text{ ml BD.}$$

CHAPTER 38

Chest Physiotherapy

Definition

Chest physiotherapy (CPT) is a technique used to **mobilize or loose secretions in the lungs** and respiratory tract. This is especially helpful for patients with large amount of secretions or ineffective cough. Chest physiotherapy consists of external mechanical maneuvers, such as chest percussion, postural drainage, vibration, to augment mobilization and clearance of airway secretions, diaphragmatic breathing with pursed-lips, coughing and controlled coughing.

Indications of Chest Physiotherapy

It is indicated for patients in whom cough is insufficient to clear thick, tenacious, or localized secretions. Examples include:

- Cystic fibrosis
- Bronchiectasis
- Atelctasis
- Lung abscess
- Neuromuscular diseases
- Pneumonias in dependent lung regions.

Contraindications of Chest Physiotherapy

- Increased ICP
- Unstable head or neck injury
- Active hemorrhage with hemodynamic instability or hemoptysis
- Recent spinal injury or injury
- Empyma
- Bronchoplueral fistula
- Rib fracture
- Fail chest
- Uncontrolled hypertension
- Anticoagulation
- Rib or vertebral fractures or osteoporosis.

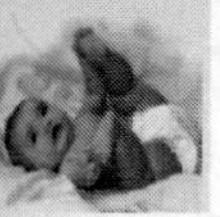

Assessment for Chest Physiotherapy

Nursing care and selection of CPT skills are based on specific assessment findings. The following are the assessment criteria:

- Check patient's vital signs. Conditions requiring CPT, such atelectasis, and pneumonia, affecting vital signs.
- Check Patient's medications. Certain medications, particularly diuretics antihypertensive cause fluid and haemodynamic changes. These decrease patient's tolerance to positional changes and postural drainage.
- Take patient's medical history; certain conditions such as increased ICP, spinal cord injuries and abdominal aneurysm resection, contra indicate the positional change to postural drainage. Thoracic trauma and chest surgeries also contraindicate percussion and vibration.
- Beware of patient's exercise tolerance.

Techniques in Chest Physiotherapy

Percussion

1. Chest percussion involves striking the chest wall over the area being drained.
2. Percussing lung areas involves the use of cupped palm to loosen pulmonary secretions so that they can be expectorated with ease.
3. Percussing with the hand held in a rigid dome-shaped position, the area over the lung lobes to be drained in struck in rhythmic pattern.
4. Usually the patient will be positioned in supine or prone and should not experience any pain.
5. Cupping is never done on bare skin or performed over surgical incisions, below the ribs, or over the spine or breasts because of the danger o tissue damage.
6. Typically, each area is percussed for 30 to 6oseconds several times a day.
7. If the patient has tenacious secretions, the area must be percussed for 3-5 minutes several times per day. Patients may learn how to percuss the anterior chest as well.

Vibration

1. In vibration, the nurse uses rhythmic contractions and relaxations of her arm and shoulder muscles while holding the patient flat on the patient's chest as the patient exhales.
2. The purpose is to help loosen respiratory secretions so that they can be expectorated with ease. Vibration (at a rate of 200 per minute) can be done for several times a day.
3. To avoid patient causing discomfort, vibration is never done over the patient's breasts, spine, sternum, and rib cage.
4. Vibration can also be taught to family members or accomplished with mechanical device.

Procedure: Percussion & Vibration

1. Instruct the patient use diaphragmatic breathing.

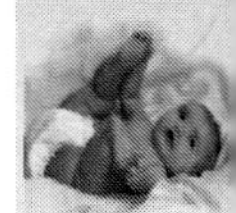

2. Position the patient in prescribed postural drainage positions. Spine should be straight to promote rib cage expansion.
3. Percuss or clap with cupped hands or chest wall for 5 minutes over each segment for 5 minutes for cystic fibrosis and 1-2 minutes for other conditions.
4. Avoid clapping over spine, liver, spleen, breast, scapula, clavicle or sternum.
5. Instruct the patient to inhale slowly and deeply. Vibrate the chest wall as the patient exhales slowly through the pursed lips.
6. Place one hand on top of the other affected over area or place one hand place one and on each side of the rib cage.
7. Tense the muscles of the hands and hands while applying moderate pressure downward and vibrate arms and hands.
8. Relieve pressure on the thorax as the patient inhales.
9. Encourage the patient cough, using abdominal muscles, after three or four vibrations.
10. Allow the patient rest several times.
11. Listen with stethoscope for changes in breath sounds.
12. Repeat the percussion and vibration cycle according to the patient's tolerance and clinical response: usually 15-30 minutes.

Postural Drainage

1. Postural drainage is the positioning techniques that drain secretions from specific segments of the lugs and bronchi into the trachea.
2. Because some patients do not require postural drainage for all lung segments, the procedure must be based on the clinical findings.
3. In postural drainage, the person is tilted or propped at an angle to help drain secretions from the lungs.
4. Also, the chest or back may be clapped with a cupped hand to help loosen secretions—the technique called chest percussion.
5. Postural drainage cannot be used for people who are:
   - unable to tolerate the position required,
   - are taking anticoagulation drugs,
   - have recently vomited up blood,
   - have had a recent rib or vertebral fracture, or
   - have severe osteoporosis.
6. Postural drainage also cannot be used for people who are unable to produce any secretions (because when this happens, further attempts at postural drainage may lower the level of oxygen in the blood).

Procedure

1. The patient's body is positioned so that the trachea is inclined downward and below the affected chest area.

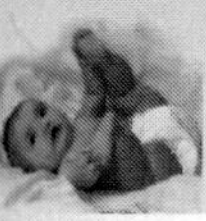

2. Postural drainage is essential in treating bronchiectasis and patients must receive physiotherapy to learn to tip themselves into a position in which the lobe to be drained is uppermost at least three times daily for 10-20 minutes.
3. The treatment is often used in conjunction with the technique for loosening secretions in the chest cavity called chest percussion.

Articles required

- Pillows
- Tilt table
- Sputum cup
- Paper tissues

Steps

1. Use specific positions so the force of gravity can assist in the removal of bronchial secretions from affected lung segments to central airways by means of coughing and suctioning.
2. The patient is positioned so that the diseased area is in a near vertical position, and gravity is used to assist the drainage of specific segment.
3. The positions assumed are determined by the location, severity, and duration of mucous obstruction.
4. The exercises are performed two to three times a day, before meals and bedtime. Each position is done for 3-15 minutes.
5. The procedure should be discontinued if tachycardia, palpitations, dyspnea, or chest occurs. The symptoms may indicate hypoxemia. Discontinue if hemoptysis occurs.
6. Bronchodilators, mucolytics agents, water, or saline may be nebulised and inhaled before postural drainage and chest percussion to reduce bronchospasm, decrease thickness of mucus and sputum, and combat edema of the bronchial walls, there by enhancing secretion removal.
7. Perform secretion removal procedures before eating.
8. Make sure patient is comfortable before the procedure starts and as comfortable as possible he or she assumes each position.
9. Auscultate the chest to determine the areas of needed drainage.
10. Encourage the patient to deep breathe and cough after spending the allotted time in each position.
11. Encourage diaphragmatic breathing through out postural drainage: this helps widen airways so secretions can be drained.

Positions

Child	
Bilateral-Apical segments	Sitting on nurse's lap, leaning slightly forward flexed over pillow.
Bilateral-middle anterior segments	Sitting on nurse's lap, leaning against nurse
Bilateral- anterior segments	Lying supine on nurse's lap, back supported with pillow.

Coughing

1. Coughing gently or making short grunting noises with the mouth slightly open will help loosen the mucus.
2. Do this periodically throughout the drainage procedure.

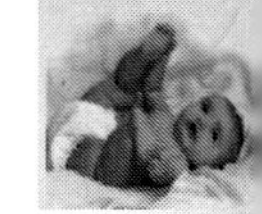

Controlled Coughing Technique

1. Controlled coughing is one of the essential techniques in good respiratory care.
2. Patient perform this maneuver after each drainage position and often throughout the day.
3. The abdominal muscles are very powerful muscles used in coughing and exhaling.
4. Inhale deeply through the nose.
5. Pause.
6. Cough 2 to 3 sharp staccato cough with proper hand/arm placement.
7. Breathe in easily through the nose.

CHAPTER 39

Nursing Care of Baby with HIV Positive Mother

Introduction

Human immunodeficiency virus infection and acquired immune deficiency syndrome (HIV/AIDS) is a disease of the human immune system caused by infection with human immunodeficiency virus (HIV). HIV is transmitted primarily via unprotected sexual intercourse (including anal and oral sex), contaminated blood transfusions, hypodermic needles, and from mother to child during pregnancy, delivery, or breastfeeding. Some bodily fluids, such as saliva and tears, do not transmit HIV.

Mother-to-child Transmission

HIV can be transmitted from mother to child during pregnancy, during delivery, or through breast milk. This is the third most common way in which HIV is transmitted globally. In the absence of treatment, the risk of transmission before or during birth is around 20% and in those who also breastfeed 35%. With appropriate treatment the risk of mother-to-child infection can be reduced to about 1%. Preventive treatment involves the mother taking antiretroviral during pregnancy and delivery, an elective caesarean section, avoiding breastfeeding, and administering antiretroviral drugs to the newborn.

Nursing Care of Baby with HIV Positive Mother

1. Use standard precautions.
2. Cut cord under cover of light gauze with a fresh blade.
3. Clean baby thoroughly of secretions.
4. Full neonatal clinical examination should be done.
5. Vitamin K should be given IM in right leg (Parent consent needed).
6. No BCG vaccination or other live vaccines should be given until baby's status is clear.
7. Give single dose of Nevprarine 2mg/kg for baby within 72 hrs of birth.
8. Baby is not given breast milk or breastfed (as there is increased risk of HIV transmission to baby). But after initiation of antiretroviral therapy exclusive breast feeding should be started.
9. Newborn infants should have a test on day 1, at least 0.5 ml EDTA, and not cord blood (this can be contaminated with maternal blood).
10. **Antiretroviral Medication:**
    a. *Monotherapy:* Most infants require this. Start the baby on AZT (Zidovudine) within 4 hours of delivery. The dose is 4 mg/kg twice daily p. o. continued for a period of 4 weeks.
    b. *Combination Therapy:* Triple therapy usually consists of AZT (Zidovudine), 3TC (Lamivudine and NVP (Nevirapine). The treatment is continued for 4 weeks.

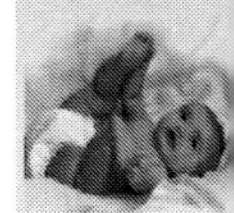

11. **Subsequent Outpatient Management**

   a. *General:* If the infant looks clinically unwell at any stage (even without a positive HIV PCR) consider measuring CD4 lymphocyte count and percentage(normal in 1st year of life 3000, 35%).

   b. *4 weeks:*

      - Only infants who have received combination ART require an appointment at 4 weeks.
      - Full clinical examination monitoring for growth and development.
      - FBC (Full Blood Count).
      - HIV PCR.

   c. *6-8 weeks:*

      - Full clinical examination monitoring for growth and development.
      - FBC to monitor for bone marrow depression.
      - HIV PCR.
      - Ensure Hepatitis B Vaccine has been given and that immunization schedule is being followed.

   d. *12 weeks:*

      - Full clinical examination monitoring for growth and development.
      - HIV PCR (0.5 ml in EDTA Bottle). If this PCR is negative then the infant is very unlikely to be infected and cotrimoxazole if previously commenced may be discontinued.
      - FBC.
      - Ensure Hepatitis B Vaccine has been given and that immunization schedule is being followed.
      - If the third PCR is negative then the infant should routinely be offered BCG vaccination.

   e. *12 months:* General clinic review.

   f. *18 months:*

      - General clinic review.
      - HIV PCR and HIV antibody. If both negative and the infant is well then discharge from clinic.

APPENDIX

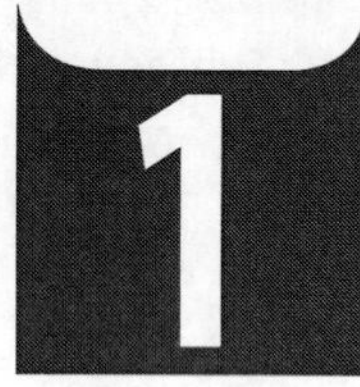

Common Drugs used in Pediatrics

Adenosine

Dosage: SVT: 0.1 mg/kg/IV/IO rapid push (max 6 mg), second dose 0.2 mg/kg/IV/IO rapid push (max 12 mg).

Indications: Supra-ventricular tachycardia.

Contraindications: 2nd and 3rd degree AV Block, sick sinus syndrome unless pacemaker is placed.

Adverse Effects

- **CNS:** Light-headedness, dizziness, arm tingling, numbness, apprehension, blurred vision, headache.
- **Eye & ENT:** Metallic taste, throat tightness.
- **Respiratory:** Dyspnea, hyperventilation, bronchospasm.
- **Cardiovascular:** Hypotension, transient bradycardia or asystole, atrial tachyarrhythmias, angina, palpitations.
- **Gastrointestinal:** Nausea.
- **Skin:** Facial and systemic flushing, sweating.

Special Nursing Considerations

- If possible, record multiple-lead rhythm strip during administration.
- Administer via central venous access if present; otherwise by IV/IO at most proximal injection site.
- Push adenosine rapidly IV/IO followed immediately by NS flush (5-10 mL).
- Theophylline is an adenosine receptor antagonist and reduces adenosine effectiveness.
- Dose need to be reduced in patients taking carbamazepine or dipyridamole and in patients with transplanted hearts.

Albumin

Dosage: 0.5-1 g/kg (10-20 mL/kg of 5% solution) IV/IO rapid infusion.

Indications: Shock, trauma, burns.

Contraindications: CHF, Severe anemia.

Adverse Effects

- **Respiratory:** Pulmonary edema (if fluid overloaded), increased respiratory rate, bronchospasm (rare allergic reaction).

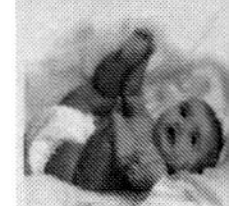

- **Cardiovascular:** Fluid overload, (can produce hypertension), hypotension, tachycardia.
- **Skin:** Rash, urticaria, flushing.
- **Miscellaneous:** Fever, hypocalcemia.

Special Nursing Considerations

- Monitor for signs of pulmonary edema. Administer slowly.
- Albumin binds calcium, so rapid infusions may decrease ionized calcium concentration, leading to hypotension.
- Albumin also binds many drugs, such as phenytoin, which may reduce free drug concentration and therapeutic effect.
- Blood product-transfusion-like reactions rarely occur.
- For IV administration, use within 4 hours of opening vial.
- 5% albumin is generally used undiluted; 25% albumin may be given undiluted or diluted in NS.

Albuterol

Dosage

- **MDI:** 4-8 puffs via inhalation q 20 minutes prn with spacer (OR ET if intubated).
- **Nebulizer:** 2.5 mg/dose (wt<20 kg) OR 5 mg/dose (wt>20 kg) via inhalation q 20 minutes prn.
- **Continuous nebulizer:** 0.5 mg/kg per hour via inhalation (max 20 mg/h).

Indications: Asthma, anaphylaxis (bronchospasm), hyperkalemia.

Contra-indications: Tachyarrhythmias, severe cardiac disease, or hypersensitivity to albuterol or adrenergic amines.

Adverse Effects

- **CNS:** Tremors, anxiety, insomnia, headache, dizziness, hallucinations.
- **Eye and ENT:** Dry nose and throat, irritation of nose and throat, bad taste.
- **Respiratory:** Wheezing, dyspnea, bronchospasm, cough (rare).
- **Cardiovascular:** Palpitations, tachycardia, systolic hypertension with wide pulse pressure, angina, hypotension, tachyarrhythmias.
- **Gastrointestinal:** Heartburn, nausea, vomiting, diarrhoea.
- **Skin:** Flushing, sweating, angio-edema.

Special Nursing Considerations

- May be combined in the same nebulizer with ipratropium bromide.
- Increased risk of tachyarrhythmias when combined with theophylline or simultaneous use of other adrenergic agents (eg. terbutaline, dopamine).

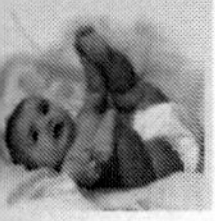

Amidarone

Dosage

- **SVT, VT (with pulses):** 5 mg/kg IV/IO load over 20-60 minutes (max 300 mg), repeat to daily max 15 mg/kg (2.2 g in adolescents).
- **Pulseless arrest (i.e, VF/pulseless VT):** 5 mg/kg IV/Io bolus (max 300 mg), repeat to daily max 15 mg/kg (2.2 g in adolescence).

  Indications: Supra-ventricular tachycardia, ventricular tachycardia, pulseless arrest.

  Contraindications: Sinus node dysfunction, second or third-degree AV block.

Adverse Effects

- **CNS:** Headache, dizziness, involuntary movements, tremors, peripheral neuropathy, malaise, fatigue, ataxia, paresthesias, syncope.
- **Respiratory:** Pulmonary fibrosis, pulmonary inflammation, ARDS.
- **Cardiovascular:** Hypotension (related to infusion rate), bradycardia, CHF, prolonged QT interval, torsades de pointes.
- **Gastrointestinal:** nausea, vomiting, diarrhoea, abdominal pain.
- **Skin:** Rash, photosensitivity, blue-gray skin discoloration, alopecia, ecchymosis, toxic epidermal necrolysis, flushing.
- **Endocrine:** Hyperthyroidism, hypothyroidism (chronic use).
- **Hematologic:** Coagulation abnormalities.

Special Nursing Considerations

- Monitor blood pressure frequently and ECG continuously.

Atropine Sulphate

Dosage

- **Bradycardia (symptomatic):**
  - 0.02 mg/kg IV/IO (min. dose 0.1 mg, max. single dose child 0.5 mg, max. single dose adolescence 1 mg), may repeat dose once, max total dose child 1 mg, max. total dose adolescence 3 mg.
  - 0.04-0.06 mg/kg ET.
- **Toxins/overdose (e.g. organophosphate, carbamate):**
  - <12 years: 0.02- 0.05 mg/kg IV/IO initially, then repeat IV/IO q20-30 minutes until muscarinic symptoms reverse.
  - >12 years: 2 mg/IV/IO initially, then 1-2 mg/IV/IO q20-30 minutes until muscarinic symptoms reverse.

Indications: Bradycardia (symptomatic), toxins/overdose (e.g. organophosphate, carbamate), rapid sequence intubation (RSI).

Contraindications: Angle-closure glaucoma, tachyarrhythmias, thryotoxicosis.

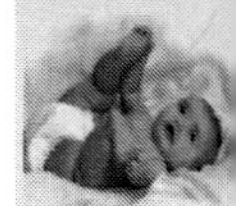

Adverse Effects

- **CNS:** Headache, dizziness, involuntary movements, confusion, psychosis, anxiety, coma, flushing, drowsiness, weakness.
- **Eye and ENT:** Blurred vision, photophobia, glaucoma, eye pain, pupil dilation, nasal congestion, dry mouth, altered taste.
- **Cardiovascular:** Tachycardia, hypotension, paradoxical bradycardia, angina, premature ventricular contractions, hypertension.
- **Gastrointestinal:** Nausea, vomiting, abdominal pain, constipation, paralytic ileus, abdominal distension.
- **Genitourinary:** Urinary retention, dysuria.
- **Skin:** Rash, urticaria, contact dermatitis, dry skin, flushing, decreased sweating.

Special Nursing Considerations

- Monitor ECG, SpO_2 and blood pressure continuously.

Calcium Chloride (10%)

Dosage: 20 mg/kg (0.2 mL/kg) IV/IO slow push during arrest, repeat prn.

Indications: Hypocalcemia, hyperkalemia, hypermagnesemia, calcium channel blocker overdose.

Contra-indications: Hypercalcemia, digitalis toxicity.

Adverse Effects

- **Cardiovascular:** Hypotension, bradycardia, asystole, shortened QT interval, heart block, and cardiac arrest.
- **Skin:** Sclerosis of peripheral veins, venous thrombosis, burn/necrosis from extravasation.
- **Electrolytes:** Hypercalcemia.

Special Nursing Considerations

- Monitor ECG continuously and blood pressure frequently.
- Central venous administration is preferred if available.
- When infusing calcium and sodium bicarbonate, flush the tubing with NS before and after infusion of each drug to avoid formation of an insoluble precipitate in the catheter lumen.

Chloral Hydrate

Dosage: 20 mg/kg oral sedation.

Indications: sedative, hypnotic.

Contra-indications: hepatic or renal disease, severe cardiac disease, gastritis.

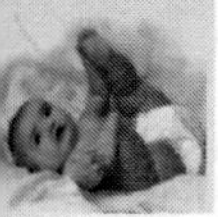

Adverse Effects

- **CNS:** excitement, delirium, mental confusion, disorientation, drowsiness.
- **Gastrointestinal:** gastric irritation, nausea, vomiting, gastric necrosis.
- **Hematologic:** leukopenia, eosinophilia.
- **Skin:** Skin irritation.

Special Nursing Considerations

- Administer syrup in half glass of water.
- Do not withdraw the drug abruptly.

Dexamethasone

Dosage: 0.6 mg/kg PO/IM/IV (max 16 mg).

Indications: Croup, Asthma.

Contra-indications: active untreated infections and fungal, viral and mycobacterial ocular infections.

Adverse Effects

- **CNS:** Depression, headache, irritability, insomnia, euphoria, seizures, psychosis, hallucinations, weakness.
- **Eye and ENT:** Fungal infections, increased intra-ocular pressure, blurred vision.
- **Cardiovascular:** Hypertension, thrombophlebitis, embolism, tachycardia, edema.
- **Gastrointestinal:** Diarrhoea, nausea, abdominal distension, pancreatitis, gastro-intestinal bleeding.
- **Musculoskeletal:** Fractures, osteoporosis.
- **Skin:** Flushing, sweating, acne, poor wound healing, ecchymosis, petechiae, hirsutism.
- **Endocrine:** Hypothalmic-pituitary-adrenal axis suppression, hyperglycaemia, sodium and fluid retention.
- **Hematologic:** Hemorrhage, thrombocytopenia.
- **Electrolytes:** Hypokalemia.

Special Nursing Considerations

- Administer by slow, direct IV injection.
- Avoid exposure to infections.
- Do not stop the drug without consultation.
- Report adverse effects.

Dextrose (Glucose)

Dosage: 0.5-1 g/kg IV/IO (D25W 2-4 mL/kg; D10W 5-10 ml/kg).

Indications: Hypoglycemia.

Contraindications: Hyperglycemia.

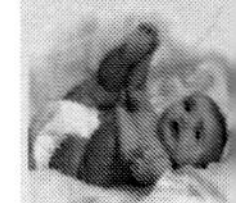

Adverse Effects

- **Skin:** Sclerosis of veins (with hypertonic glucose concentrations).
- **Endocrine:** Hyperglycemia, hyperosmolarity.

Special Nursing Considerations

- Do not administer routinely during resuscitation unless hypoglycaemia is documented.
- Administer slowly.
- Monitor patient for fluid overload, blood sugars.
- Inspect injection site frequently.

Diazepam

Dosage

- **Sedative/muscle relaxant:** 0.04-0.2 mg/kg/dose q2-4 hr; max. dose: 0.6 mg/kg within an 8-hr period.
- **Status epilepticus:** 0.2-0.5mg/kg IV q15-30 mins; may be repeated 4-8 hourly.

Indications: anxiety, skeletal muscle spasm, status epilepticus.

Contra-indications: Myasthenia gravis, severe respiratory insufficiency, severe hepatic failure, sleep apnea syndrome.

Adverse Effects

- **CNS:** Sedation, clamminess, sweating, headache, vertigo, floating feeling, dizziness, lethargy, confusion, light-headedness.
- **Gastro-intestinal:** Nausea, vomiting.
- **Cardiovascular:** Palpitation, changed BP.
- **Respiratory:** Slow and shallow respiration.
- **Local:** injection site reactions.

Special Nursing Considerations

- Do not use small veins for IV injection.
- Monitor vital signs of the patient during IV administration.
- Maintain patients receiving IV injection in bed for 3 hours.

Diphenhydramine

Dosage: 1-2 mg/kg IV/IO/IM q4-6 hours (max. single dose 50 mg).

Indications: Anaphylactic shock.

Contraindications: concurrent use of MAO inhibitor use, acute asthma attacks, GI or urinary obstruction.

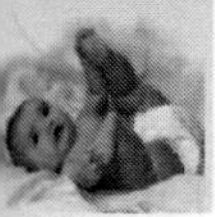

Adverse Effects

- **CNS:** Dizziness, drowsiness, poor coordination, fatigue, anxiety, euphoria, confusion, paresthesia, neuritis, seizures, dystonic reaction, hallucinations, sedation.
- **Eye and ENT:** Blurred vision, pupil dilation, tinnitus, nasal stuffiness, dry nose/mouth/throat.
- **Cardiovascular:** Hypotension, palpitations, tachycardia.
- **Respiratory:** Chest tightness.
- **Gastrointestinal:** Nausea, vomiting, diarrhoea.
- **Genitourinary:** Urinary retention, dysuria, frequency.
- **Skin:** Photosensitivity, rash.
- **Hematologic:** Thrombocytopenia, agranulocytosis, haemolytic anemia.
- **Miscellaneous:** Anaphylaxis.

Special Nursing Considerations

- Monitor SpO_2 continuously and blood pressure frequently.

Dobutamine

Dosage: 2-20 mcg/kg per minute IV/IO infusion; titrate to desired effect.

Indications: congestive heart failure, cardiogenic shock, ventricular dysfunction.

Contraindications: idiopathic hypertrophic sub-aortic stenosis (IHSS).

Adverse Effects

- **CNS:** Anxiety, headache, dizziness.
- **Cardiovascular:** Hypotension, hypertension, palpitations, tachyarrhythmia, premature ventricular contractions, angina.
- **Gastrointestinal:** Nausea, vomiting, mucositis.
- **Hematologic:** Thrombocytopenia.

Special Nursing Considerations

- Monitor ECG continuously and blood pressure frequently.
- May be given via peripheral IV.
- Drug is inactivated in alkaline solutions.

Dopamine

Dosage: 2-20 mcg/kg per minute IV/IO infusion; titrate to desired effect.

Indications: cardiogenic shock including ventricular dysfunction, distributive shock.

Contraindications: Pheochromocytoma, tachyarrhythmias, hypovolemia.

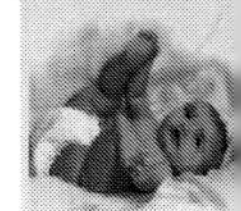

Adverse Effects

CNS: Headache.

Respiratory: Dyspnea.

Cardiovascular: Palpitations, premature ventricular contractions, SVT, VT, hypertension, peripheral vasoconstriction.

Gastrointestinal: Nausea, vomiting, diarrhoea.

Genitourinary: Acute renal failure.

Skin: Local necrosis (with infiltration), gangrene.

Special Nursing Considerations

- Monitor ECG continuously and blood pressure frequently.
- High infusion rates (>20 mcg/kg/min) produce peripheral, renal and splanchnic vasoconstriction and ischemia; if infusion dose >20 mcg/kg/min is required, consider addition of alternative adrenergic agent (e.g. epinephrine/nor-epinephrine).
- Do not mix with sodium bicarbonate.
- Tissue ischemia and necrosis may result if IV infiltration occurs. Infiltration with phentolamine may reduce local effect of dopamine.
- Central venous administration is preferred.
- Inactivated in alkaline solutions.

Epinephrine

Dosage

- **Pulseless arrest, bradycardia (symptomatic):** 0.01 mg/kg (0.1 mL/kg of 1:10,000 standard concentrations) IV/IO q3-5 minutes (max. single dose 1 mg) 0.1 mg/kg (0.1 mL/kg of 1:1000 high concentrations) ET q 3-5 minutes.
- Hypotensive shock: 0.1-1 mcg/kg per minute IV/IO infusion (consider high doses if needed).
- Anaphylaxis.

IM autoinjector 0.3 mg (for patient weighing >30 kg) or IM junior auto-injector 0.15 mg (for patient weighing 10-30 kg).

0.01 mg/kg (0.01 mL/kg of 1:1000 high concentrations) IM q15 minutes prn (max single dose 0.3 mg).

0.01 mg/kg (0.01 mL/kg of 1:10,000 standard concentrations) IV/IO q3-5 minutes (max single dose 1 mg) if hypotensive.

0.1-1 mcg/kg per minute IV/IO infusion if hypotension persists despite fluids and IM injection.

- **Asthma:** 0.01 mg/kg (0.01 mL/kg) 1:1000 subcutaneously q15 minutes (max 0.3 mg or 0.3 mL).
- **Croup:** 0.25-0.5 mg racemic solution (2.25%) mixed in 3mL NS via inhalation.

3 mL of 1:1000 epinephrine mixed with 3 mL NS (which yields 0.25 mL racemic epinephrine solution via inhalation).

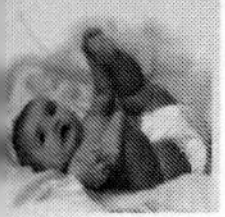

Indications: Pulseless arrest, bradycardia (symptomatic), Hypotensive shock, Anaphylaxis, Asthma, Croup.

Contraindications: Coccaine-induced VT.

Adverse Effects

- **CNS:** Tremors, anxiety, insomnia, headache, dizziness, weakness, drowsiness, confusion, hallucinations, intracranial hemorrhage.
- **Respiratory:** Dyspnea.
- **Cardio-vascular:** Arrhythmias, palpitations, tachycardia, hypertension, ST-segment elevation, post-resuscitation myocardial dysfunction.
- **Gastro-intestinal:** Nausea, vomiting.
- **Genito-urinary:** Renal vascular ischemia.
- **Endocrine:** Hyperglycaemia, post-resuscitation hyper-adrenergic state.
- **Electrolytes:** Hypokalemia.

Special Nursing Considerations

- Monitor ECG, SpO_2 continuously and blood pressure frequently.
- High doses produce vasoconstriction and may compromise organ perfusion.
- Low doses may increase cardiac output with redirection of blood flow to skeletal muscles, producing renal and splanchnic blood flow.
- Myocardial O_2 requirements are increased.
- Tissue ischemia and necrosis may result if IV infiltration occurs. Infiltration with phentolamine may reduce local toxic effect of epinephrine.
- Central venous access si preferred for administration.
- Catecholamines are inactivated in alkaline solutions.
- Observe for atleast 2 hours after croup treatment for 'rebound' (i.e. recurrence of stridor).
- When give IM for treatment of anaphylaxis, thigh is preferred site than deltoid muscle.

Etomidate

Dosage: 0.2-0.4 mg/kg IV/IO infused over 30-60 seconds (max 20 mg) will produce rapid sedation that lasts for 10-15 minutes.

Indications: Rapid-sequence intubation (RSI).

Contraindications: Known adrenal insufficiency, history of focal seizure disorders.

Adverse Effects

- **Respiratory:** Hypoventilation or hyperventilation.
- **Cardiovascular:** Hypotension or hypertension, tachycardia.
- **Gastrointestinal:** Nausea, vomiting on emergence from anaesthesia, myoclonic activity (coughing, hiccups).

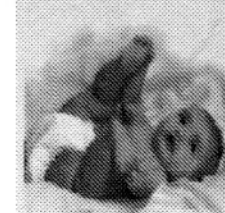

- **Endocrine:** Adrenal suppression.
- **Miscellaneous:** Myoclonus, uncontrolled eye movements, pain at injection site.

Special Nursing Considerations

- Produces rapid sedation with minimal cardio-vascular or respiratory depression.
- Because the drug may cause possible adrenal suppression, should not be used to maintain sedation after intubation.
- Use of benzodiazepines or opioids may decrease myoclonus.

Fentanyl

Dosage: 1-2 mcg/kg/dose I; 1 mcg/kg/hr IV infusion.

Indications: Sedation, pain relief, preoperative medication, adjunct to anaesthesia.

Contraindications: Raised ICP, acute bronchial asthma, upper airway obstruction, hepatic or renal problems.

Adverse Effects

- **CNS:** dizziness, sedation, drowsiness.
- **Cardiovascular:** palpitation, increase or decrease BP, circulatory depression, cardiac arrest, shock.
- **Respiratory:** slow, shallow respiration, apnea, laryngospasm.
- **Eye:** impaired visual acuity, nausea.
- **Gastrointestinal:** loss of appetite, constipation.
- **Genitourinary:** oliguria, urinary retention.

Special Nursing Considerations

- Monitor vital signs of the patient before, during and after the administration.
- Assess neurologic status of the patient.
- Administer IV injection slowly over 5-10 minutes.

Furosemide (Lasix)

Dosage: Neonate: 0.5-1 mg/kg/dose q8-24 hr IV/IM; max dose: 2 mg/kg/dose.

Infant and child: 1-2 mg/kg/dose 6-12 hr IV/IM; max dose: 6 mg/kg/dose.

Indications: Pulmonary edema, Fluid overload.

Contra-indications: anuria, hepatic coma.

Adverse Effects

- **CNS:** Headache, fatigue, weakness, vertigo, paresthesias.
- **Eye and ENT:** Hearing loss, tinnitus, blurred vision, dry oral mouth, oral irritation.

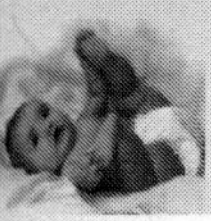

- **Cardiovascular:** Orthostatic hypotension, angina, ECG changes from electrolyte abnormalities, circulatory collapse.
- **Gastrointestinal:** Nausea, vomiting, diarrhoea, abdominal cramps, gastric irritation, pancreatitis.
- **Genitourinary:** Polyuria, renal failure, glycosuria.
- **Musculoskeletal:** Muscle cramps, stiffness.
- **Skin:** Pruritis, purpura, Stevans_johnson syndrome, sweating, photosensitivity, urticaria.
- **Endocrine:** Hyperglycemia.
- **Hematology:** Thrombocytopenia, agranulocytosis, leukopenia, naemia, neutropenia.
- **Electrolyte disturbances:** Hypokalemia, Hypochloremia, Hypomagnesemia, Hyperurecemia, Hypocalcemia, Hyponatremia.
- **Miscellaneous:** Metabolic alkalosis.

Special Nursing Considerations

- Monitor blood pressure frequently.
- Monitor serum creatinine, BUN, and electrolytes, especially potassium. Hypokalemia may be significant and requires close monitoring and replacement therapy.

Hydrocortisone

Dosage: 2 mg/kg IV bolus (max 100 mg).

Indications: Adrenal insufficiency.

Contraindications: Presence of infections, kidney or liver disease, hypothyroidism, thrombophlebitis, diabetes mellitus, convulsive disorders.

Adverse Effects

- **CNS:** Depression, headache, mood changes.
- **Eye and ENT:** Fungal infections, increased intra-ocular pressure, blurred vision.
- **Cardiovascular:** Hypertension.
- **Gastrointeestinal:** Diarrhoea, nausea, abdominal distension, peptic ulcer.
- **Musculoskeletal:** Fractures, osteoporosis, weakness.
- **Skin:** Flushing, sweating, thrombophlebitis, edema, acne, poor wound healing, ecchymosis, petechiae, pruritis.
- **Endocrine:** Hyperglycemia, suppression of hypothalamic-pituitary axis.
- **Miscellaneous:** increased risk of infection.

Special Nursing Considerations

- Inject the drug slowly, directly or dilute in normal saline or D5W.
- Give the drug exactly as prescribed. Do not stop abruptly.
- Monitor the patient for unusual weight gain, swelling of lower extremities, muscle weakness, black or tarry stools, vomiting of blood, epigastric burning, puffing of face, menstrual irregulations, fever, prolonged sore throat, cold or other infection, worsening of symptoms.

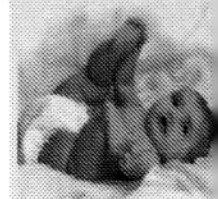

Ibuprofen

Dosage

- **Analgesic/antipyretic:** 5-10 mg/kg/dose q6-8 hr PO, max dose: 40 mg/kg/24 hr.
- **Analgesic:** 400-800 mg/dose q 4-6 hr IV; max dose: 3200 mg/24 hr.
- **Antipyretic:** 400 mg/dose q4-6 hr or 100-200 mg/dose 4 hr IV; max dose: 3200 mg/24 hr .
- **Closure of ductus arteriosus:** < 32 week of gestation and 0.5-1.5 kg : 10 mg/kg/dose IV x 1 followed by two doses of 5 mg/kg/dose each, after 24 hr and 48 hr.

Indications

- Relief of mild to moderate pain.
- Fever reduction.
- Closure of ductus arteriosus.

Contra-indications: Active GI bleed and ulcer disease; cardio-vascular dysfunction, hypertension.

Adverse Effects

- **CNS:** headache, dizziness, insomnia, somnolence.
- **Cardiovascular:** hypertension.
- **Respiratory:** Dyspnea, hemoptysis, pharyngitis, bronchospasm, rhinitis.
- **Gastrointestinal:** Nausea, dyspepsia, GI pain, constipation.
- **Eye:** Ocular problems.
- **Hematologic:** granulocytopenia, anemia, inhibit platelet aggregation, bleeding.
- **Skin:** Rashes.

Special Nursing Considerations

- Administer drug with food or after meals if GI upset occurs.
- Arrange for periodic ophthalmologic examination. Discontinue drug if eye changes, symptoms of liver or renal dysfunction appears.
- Institute emergency procedures if overdose occurs; gastric lavage, induction of emesis, supportive therapy.

Ipratropium Bromide

Dosage: 250-500 mcg via inhalation q20 minutes prn X 3 doses.

Indications: Asthma.

Contraindications: soy or peanut allergy, atropine hypersensitivity.

Adverse Effects

- **CNS:** Anxiety, dizziness, headache, nervousness.

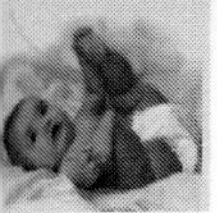

- **Eye and ENT:** Dry mouth, blurred vision (pupil dilation).
- **Respiratory:** Cough, worsening bronchospasm.
- **Cardiovascular:** Palpitations.
- **Gastrointestinal:** Nausea, vomiting, abdominal cramps.
- **Skin:** Rash.

Special Nursing Considerations

Lidocaine

Dosage: 1 mg/kg IV/IO bolus.

- **Maintenance:** 20-50 mcg/kg per minute IV/IO infusion (repeat bolus dose if infusion initiated >15 minutes after initial bolus).
- 2-3 mg/kg ET.

  Indications: VF/pulseless VT, wide-complex tachycardia (with pulses), Rapid sequence intubation (RSI)

  Contraindications: Wide-complex ventricular escape beats associated with bradycardia.

Adverse Effects

- **CNS:** Seizures (high concentrations), headache, dizziness, involuntary movement, confusion, tremor, drowsiness, euphoria.
- **Eye and ENT:** Tinnitus, blurred vision.
- **Cardio-vascular:** Hypotension, myocardial depression, bradycardia, heart block, arrhythmias, cardiac arrest.
- **Respiratory:** Dyspnea, respiratory depression or arrest.
- **Gastro-intestinal:** Nausea, vomiting.
- **Skin:** Rash, urticaria, edema, swelling, phlebitis at IV site.

Special Nursing Considerations

- Monitor ECG continuously and blood pressure frequently.
- High plasma concentration may cause myocardial and circulatory depression and CNS complications (seizures)
- Drug decreases ICP and IOP response during laryngoscopy.

Loperamide

Dosage

- **Active diarrhoea:** Initial doses within first 24-hrs: 2-5 yr (13-20 kg)- 1 mg PO TID; 6-8 yr (20-30 kg) – 2 mg PO BID; 9-12 yr (> 30 kg) – 2 mg PO TID; max single dose: 2 mg; follow initial dose with 0.1 mg/kg/dose after each loose stool (not to exceed aforementioned initial doses).
- **Chronic diarrhoea:** 0.08-0.24 mg/kg/24 hr ÷ BID-TID; max dose: 2mg/dose.

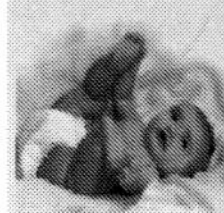

Indications: Control and symptomatic relief of acute nonspecific diarrhoea and chronic diarrhoea associated with inflammatory bowel disease.

Contraindications: acute dysentery, acute ulcerative colitis, bacterial enterocolitis caused by salmonella, shigella, campylobacter and c.difficile, abdominal pain in the absence of diarrhoea.

Adverse Effects

- **CNS:** Tiredness, drowsiness, dizziness, CNS depression.
- **Gastro-intestinal:** abdominal pain, distension or discomfort, constipation, dry mouth, nausea.

Special Nursing Considerations

- Discontinue drug if improvement is not seen within 48 hours.
- Do not exceed prescribed or recommended dose.
- Keep narcotic antagonist naloxone for CNS depression.

Lorazepam

Dosage

- **Anxiolytic/sedation:** 0.05 mg/kg/dose q4-8 hourly; max. dose 2 mg/dose.
- **Status epilepticus:** 0.05-0.1 mg/kg/dose IV over 2-5 min.; may repeat 0.05 mg/kg x 1 in 10-15 minutes.

  Indications: anxiety, sedation, status epilepticus.

  Contra-indications: narrow-angle glaucoma, severe hypotension.

Adverse Effects

- **CNS:** Drowsiness, sedation, depression, lethargy, apathy, fatigue, light-headedness, disorientation, anger, hostility, emotional upset, crying.
- **Respiratory:** Respiratory depression.
- **Cardiovascular:** Hypotension.
- **Gastrointestinal:** Constipation, diarrhoea, dry mouth, nausea.
- **Hematologic:** Rash.

Special Nursing Considerations

- Protect drug from light and refrigerate the solution.
- Use with caution when administering with other narcotic analgesics.
- Monitor vital signs of the patients.
- Maintain patients receiving IV injection in bed for 3 hours.

Magnesium Sulphate

Dosage: 25-50 mg/kg IV/IO bolus (max 2 g) (pulseless VT) OR over 10-20 minutes (VT with pulses) OR slow infusion over 15-30 minutes (status asthmaticus).

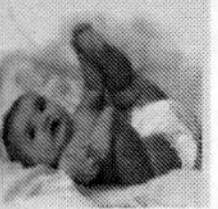

Indications: Asthma (refractory status asthmaticus), torsades de pointers, hypomagnesemia).

Contra-indications: Renal failure.

Adverse Effects

- **CNS:** Confusion, sedation, depressed reflexes, flaccid paralysis, weakness.
- **Respiratory:** Respiratory depression.
- **Cardiovascular:** Hypotension, bradycardia, heart block, cardiac arrest.
- **Gastrointestinal:** Nausea, vomiting.
- **Musculoskeletal:** Cramps.
- **Skin:** Flushing, sweating.
- **Electrolytes:** Hypermagnesemia.

Special Nursing Considerations

- Monitor ECG, SpO_2 continuously and blood pressure frequently.
- Rapid bolus may cause severe hypotension and bradycardia.
- Have calcium chloride (or calcium gluconate) available if needed to reverse magnesium toxicity.

Methylprednisolone

Dosage

- **Load:** 2 mg/kg IV/IO/IM (max 60 mg); only use acetate salt IM.
- **Maintenance:** 0.5 mg/kg IV/IO q6hours (max 120mg/day).

Indications: Asthma (status athmaticus), anaphylactic shock.

Contra-indications: GI obstruction, seizure disorder, pheochromocytoma, or in patient receiving drugs likely to cause extra-pyramidal symptoms (EPS).

Adverse Effects

- **CNS:** Depression, headache, mood changes, weakness.
- **Cardiovascular:** Hypertension.
- **Gastrointestinal:** Hemorrhage, diarrhoea, nausea, abdominal distension, pancreatitis, peptic ulcer.
- **Musculoskeletal:** Fractures, osteoporosis, arthralgia.
- **Endocrine:** Hyperglycemia.
- **Hematologic:** Transient leukocytosis.
- **Miscellaneous:** Anaphylaxis.

Special Nursing Considerations

- Inject the drug slowly, directly or dilute in normal saline or D5W.
- Give the drug exactly as prescribed. Do not stop abruptly.

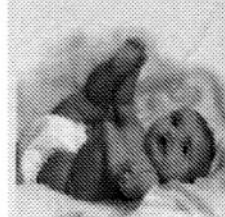

- Monitor the patient for unusual weight gain, swelling of lower extremities, muscle weakness, black or tarry stools, vomiting of blood, epigastric burning, puffing of face, menstrual irregulations, fever, prolonged sore throat, cold or other infection, worsening of symptoms.

Midazolam

Dosage: 0.1-0.3 mg/kg IV, effects lasts 1-2 hour. Alternatively 0.15-0.2 mg/kg IV loading; 1-3 mcg/kg/min.

Indications: sedation, anaesthesia, painful procedures, artificial ventilation.

Contra-indications: hypersensitivity, acute narrow angle glaucoma, shock.

Adverse Effects

- **Respiratory:** Respiratory depression.
- **Cardiovascular:** Hypotension, bradycardia.

Special Nursing Considerations

- Monitor vital signs of the patients.
- Maintain patients receiving IV injection in bed for 3 hours.
- Effects can be reversed by flumazenil.

Milrinone

Dosage: loading dose: 50 mcg/kg IV/IO over 10-60 minutes followed by 0.25-0.75 mcg/kg per minute IV/IO infusion.

Indications: Myocardial dysfunction and increased SVR/PVR.

Contra-indications: severe aortic stenosis, severe pulmonary stenosis, acute MI.

Adverse Effects

- **CNS:** Headache, tremor.
- **Cardiovascular:** Hypotension, ventricular arrhythmias, angina.
- **Gastrointestinal:** Nausea, vomiting, abdominal pain, hepatotoxicity, jaundice.
- **Hematologic:** Thrombocytopenia.
- **Electrolytes:** Hypokalemia.

Special Nursing Considerations

- Monitor ECG continuously and blood pressure frequently.
- Monitor platelet count.
- Hypovolemia may worsen hypotensive effects.
- May accumulate in renal failure and in patients with low cardiac output.
- Avoid in patients with ventricular outflow tract.
- Use of longer infusion time to administer loading dose reduces the risk of hypotension.

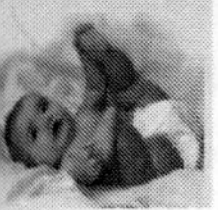

Morphine

Dosage: 0.1-0.2 mg/kg IV bolus, repeat 4-6 min.

Indications: Pain relief, relieves dyspnea of left ventricular failure and pulmonary edema, pre-anesthetic medication.

Contraindications: Respiratory depression, GI obstruction, acute and severe asthma, liver or renal problems.

Adverse Effects

- **CNS:** dizziness, sedation, drowsiness.
- **Cardiovascular:** circulatory depression, cardiac arrest, shock.
- **Respiratory:** apnea, respiratory depression, respiratory arrest.
- **Gastrointestinal:** nausea, loss of appetite, constipation.
- **Eye:** impaired visual acuity.
- **Genitourinary:** oliguria, urinary retention.

Special Nursing Considerations

- Monitor vital signs of the patient before, during and after the administration.
- Assess neurologic status of the patient.
- Dilute and administer IV slowly over 15-30 minutes.

Naloxone

Dosage

- Total reversal required (for narcotic toxicity secondary to overdose): 0.1 mg/kg IV/IO/IM/ Subcutaneous bolus q2 minutes prn (max 2 mg).
- Total reversal not required (e.g. for respiratory depression associated with therapeutic narcotic use): 1-5 mcg/kg IV/IO/IM/Subcutaneous, titrated to desired effect.
- Maintain reversal: 0.002 to 0.16 mg/kg per hour IV/IO infusion.

Indications: Narcotic (opiate reversal).

Contra-indications: allergy to narcotic antagonists.

Adverse Effects

- **CNS:** Seizures, drowsiness, nervousness.
- **Respiratory:** Hyperpnea, pulmonary edema.
- **Cardiovascular:** VF/VT, tachycardia, hypertension, asystole.
- **Gastrointestinal:** nausea, vomiting.

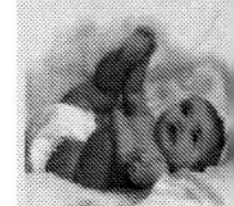

Special Nursing Considerations

- Monitor ECG and SpO_2 continuously and blood pressure frequently.
- Repeat dosing is often required because half-life of naloxone is often shorter than the half-life of opioid being reversed.
- Administration to newborns of addicted mothers may precipitate seizures or other withdrawal symptoms.
- In overdose patients, establish effective assisted ventilation before administration of naloxone to avoid excessive sympathetic nervous system stimulation.
- Drug exerts some analgesic effects.

Nifedipine

Dosage

- Hypertensive urgency: 0.25-0.5 mg/kg/dose q4-6 hr PRN PO/SL; max dose 10 mg/dose or 1-2 mg/kg/24 hr.
- Hypertension: sustained release: start with 0.25-0.5 mg/kg/24 hr ÷ 12-24 hr. May increase to max dose: 3 mg/kg/24 hr upto 120 mg/24 hr.
- Hypertrophic cardiomyopathy: 0.6-0.9 mg/kg/24 hr ÷ 6-8 hr PO/SL.

Indications: Hypertension, angina pectoris, stable angina.

Contra-indications: allergy to nifedipine.

Adverse Effects

- **CNS:** Dizziness, light headedness, headache, asthenia, nervousness.
- **Cardiovascular:** Peripheral edema, angina, bradycardia, AV block, severe hypotension. Tachycardia, palpitations.
- **Gastrointestinal:** nausea, diarrhoea, constipation.
- **Skin:** Flushing, rash.

Special Nursing Consideration

- Monitor cardiac rhythm, BP and urinary output regularly.
- Ensure that patients do not chew or divide sustained-release tablets.
- Do not administer with grapefruit juice.
- Protect drug from light and moisture.

Nitroglycerine

Dosage: Initiate at 0.25-0.5 mcg/kg per minute IV/IO infusion, titrate by 1 mcg/kg per minute q 15-20 minutes as tolerated, typical dose range 1-5 mcg/kg per minute (max dose 10 mcg/kg per minute).

In adolescents, start with 5-10 mcg per minute (not per kilogram per minute) and increase to max 200 mcg per minute.

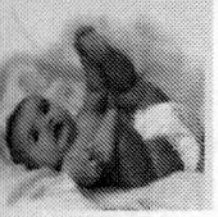

Indications: Congestive heart failure, cardiogenic shock.

Contraindications: Glaucoma, sever anaemia.

Adverse Effects

- **CNS:** Headache, dizziness.
- **Respiratory:** Hypoxemia .
- **Cardiovascular:** Postural hypotension, tachycardia, cardiac arrest, syncope paradoxical bradycardia
- **Skin:** Flushing, pallor, sweating.

Special Nursing Considerations

- Monitor ECG continuously and blood pressure frequently.
- May cause hypotension, especially in hypovolemic patients.

Nitroprusside

Dosage: 0.3-1 mcg/kg/per minute initial dose; then titrate upto 8 mcg/kg per minute as needed.

Indications: Cardiogenic shock (i.e. associated with high SVR), severe hypertension.

Contraindications: Decreased cerebral perfusion, compensatory hypertension (increased ICP).

Adverse Effects

- **CNS:** Seizures (thiocyanate toxicity), dizziness, headache, agitation, decreased reflexes, restlessness.
- **Cardiovascular:** Hypotension, bradycardia, tachycardia.
- **Gastrointestinal:** nausea, vomiting, abdominal cramps.
- **Endocrine:** hypothyroidism.
- **Miscellaneous:** Cyanide and thiocyanate toxicity.

Special Nursing Considerations

- Use special administration tubing or wrap drug reservoir in aluminium foil or another opaque material to protect it from deterioration with exposure to light.
- Use solution immediately after preparation.
- Freshly prepared solution may have a very faint brownish tint without change in drug potency.
- May react with a variety of substances to form highly colored reaction products.

Norepinephrine

Dosage: 0.1-2 mcg/kg per minute IV/IO infusion; titrate to desired effect.

Indications: Hypotensive (usually distributive) shock (i.e. low SVR and fluid refractory).

Contraindications: Hypovolemia, profound hypoxia or hypercarbia, mesenteric or peripheral vascular thrombosis.

Adverse Effects

- **CNS:** Headache, anxiety.
- **Respiratory:** Respiratory distress.
- **Cardiovascular:** Hypertension, tachycardia, bradycardia, arrhythmias.
- **Genitourinary:** Renal failure.
- **Skin:** Local necrosis (infiltration).

Special Nursing Considerations

- Monitor ECG continuously and blood pressure frequently.
- May produce hypertension, organ ischemia or arrhythmias.
- Tissue infiltration may produce sever ischemia and necrosis.
- Do not mix with sodium bicarbonate.
- Ideally should be administered via central venous catheter.
- Drug is inactivated in alkaline solutions.

Paracetamol/Acetaminophen

Dosage: Neonate: 10-15 mg/kg/dose PO/PR q6-8 hr; Pediatric: 10-15 mg/kg/dose PO/PR/IV q4-6 hr: max dose: 90 mg/kg/24 hr.

Indications: Analgesic- antipyretic effect.

Contraindications: allergy to acetaminophen; caution use in hepatic dysfucntion.

Adverse Effects

- **CNS:** Headache.
- **Cardiovascular:** chest pain, dyspnea.
- **Gastrointestinal:** Hepatic toxicity and failure, jaundice, nausea, vomiting, constipation.
- Hyper-sensitivity reactions

Special Nursing Considerations

- Do not exceed the recommended dose.
- Administer with food if GI upset is reported.

Phenytoin

Dosage

- **Status epilepticus:** loading- 15-20 mg/kg IV; max dose: 1500 mg/24 hr.
- **Maintenance for seizure disorders:** Neonate: start with 5 mg/kg/24 hr PO/IV ÷ q12 hr; usual range 5-8 mg/kg/24 hr PO/IV ÷ q8-12 hr. Infant/child: start with 5 mg/kg/24 hr ÷ BID-TID PO/IV; usual dose range (doses divided BID-TID):
  - 6 mo-3 yr: 8-10 mg/kg/24 hr

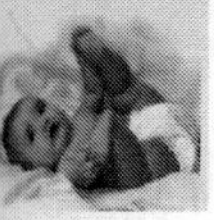

- 4-6 yr: 7.5-9 mg/kg/24 hr
- 7-9 yr: 7-8 mg/kg/24 hr
- 10-16 yr: 6-7 mg/kg/24 hr

Indications

- Control of grand mal (tonic-clonic) and psychomotor seizures.
- Prevention and treatment of seizures occurring during or following neurosurgery.
- Control of status epilepticus of grand mal type.

Contra-indications: Heart block, sinus bradycardia.

Adverse Effects

- **CNS:** Nystagmus, ataxia, dysarthria, slurred speech, mental consuion, dizziness, drowsiness, insomnia, transient nervousness, motor twitching, fatigue, irritability, depression, numbness, tremors, headache.
- **Gastrointestinal:** Nausea, gingival hyperplasia.
- **Hematologic:** Blood dyscrasia, lymphadenopathy.
- **Skin:** dermatitis, Stevans-Johnsons syndrome.

Special Nursing Considerations

- Monitor patient's cardiac rhythm and BP frequently during IV infusion.
- Administer IV slowly to prevent severe hypotension.
- Monitor injection sites carefully for phlebitis.
- Administer oral drug with food to enhance absorption and prevent GI upset.
- Administer drug exactly as advised. Do not change dose, stop abruptly or replace with other anti-epileptic agent.
- Maintain good oral hygiene (regular brushing and flossing) to prevent gum disease. Arrange for regular dental check-ups.
- Monitor renal function, liver function, blood counts regularly.

Procainamide

Dosage: 15 mg. kg IV/IO load over 30-60 minutes (do not use routinely with amidarone).

Indications: SVT, atrial flutter, VT (with pulses).

Contraindications: Myasthenia gravis, complete heart block, Systemic lupus erythematous, torsades de pointus.

Adverse Effects

- **CNS:** Headache, dizziness, confusion, psychosis, restlessness, irritability, weakness.
- **CV:** Hypotension, negative inotropic effects, prolonged QT interval, torsades de pointes, heart block, cardiac arrest.
- **Gastrointestinal:** Nausea, vomiting, diarrhea, hepatomegaly.

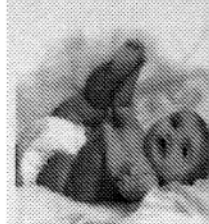

- **Skin:** Rash, urticaria, edema, swelling, pruritus, flushing.
- **Hematology:** Systemic lupus erythematous syndrome, agranulocytosis, thrombocytopenia, neutropenia, haemolytic anemia.

Special Nursing Considerations

- Monitor ECG continuously with focus on T interval, and monitor blood pressure frequently.
- Risk of hypotension and negative inotropic effects increases with rapid administration.
- Administration in combination with amidarone (or other agents that prolong QT interval) is not recommended.
- Reduce dose for patients with poor renal or cardiac function.
- Monitor procainamide and N-acetyl procainamide (NAPA) concentrations.

Prostaglandin E1 (PGE1)

Dosage: 0.05-0.1 mcg/kg per minute IV/IO infusion initially, then 0.01-0.05 mcg/kg per minute IV/IO.

Indications: Ductal-dependent congenital heart disease such as cyanotic defects (e.g. transposition of great vessels, tricuspid atresia, tetralogy of Fallot); left heart or ascending aortic obstructive lesions (e.g. hypoplastic left heart syndrome, critical aortic stenosis, coarctation of aorta, interrupted aortic arch).

Contraindications: respiratory distress syndrome, conditions predisposing to priapism.

Adverse Effects

- **CNS:** Seizures, jitteriness.
- **Respiratory:** Apnea, bronchospasm.
- **Cardiovascular:** Vasodilation, hypotension, bradycardia, tachycardia, cardiac arrest.
- **Gastrointestinal:** Gastric outlet obstruction, diarrhea.
- **Genitourinary:** Renal failure.
- **Musculoskeletal:** Cortical proliferation of long bones (after prolonged treatment, seen as periosteal new bone formation on X-ray).
- **Skin:** Flushing, edema, urticaria.
- **Endocrine:** Hypoglycemia.
- **Hematology:** Disseminated intravascular coagulation, leukocytosis, hemorrhage, thrombocytopenia
- **Electrolyte disturbances:** Hypocalcemia.
- **Miscellaneous:** Fever.

Special Nursing Considerations

- Adverse effects are dose-related.
- Extravasation may cause tissue sloughing and necrosis.
- Drug may also be given via umbilical arterial catheter positioned near ductus arteriosus.
- PGE1 should be refrigerated until administered.

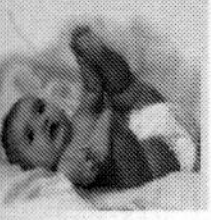

Sodium Bicarbonate

Dosage

- **Metabolic acidosis (severe), hyperkalemia:** 1 mEq/kg IV/IO slow bolus.
- **Sodium channel blocker overdose (e.g. tricylic antidepressant):** 1-2 mEq/kg IV bolus until serum pH is >7.45 (7.50-7.55 for severe poisoning) followed by IV/IO infusion of 150 mEq NaHCO3/L solution titrated to maintain alkalosis.

Indications: Metabolic acidosis (severe), hyperkalemia, Sodium channel blocker overdose (e.g. tricyclic antidepressant).

Contraindications: respiratory alkalosis, hypochloremia, inadequate ventilation during cardiac arrest

Adverse Effects

- **CNS:** Irritability, headache, confusion, stimulation, tremors, hyper-reflexia, tetany, seizures, weakness.
- **Respiratory:** Respiratory depression, apnea.
- **Cardiovascular:** Arrhythmia, hypotension, cardiac arrest.
- **Gastrointestinal:** Abdominal distension, paralytic ileus.
- **Genitourinary:** Renal calculi.
- **Skin:** Cyanosis, edema, sclerosis/necrosis (infiltration), vasodilation.
- **Electrolyte imbalances:** Hypernatremia, Hyperosmolarity, Hypocalcemia, Hypokalemia.

Special Nursing Considerations

Monitor SpO_2, and ECG continuously.

Monitor ABG.

Ensure adequate ventilation because buffering action produces CO_2, which crosses blood-brain-barrier and cell membranes more rapidly than HCO_3, If ventilation is inadequate, increased CO_2 may result in transient paradoxical CSF and intracellular acidosis.

Drug may inactivate catecholamines.

By increasing pH, will produce a decrease in serum potassium and ionized calcium concentrations.

- When combined with calcium salts, will precipitate into insoluble calcium carbonate crystals that may obstruct the IV catheter or tubing.
- Routine administration is not recommended in cardiac arrest.
- Drug should not be administered via endo-tracheal route.
- Irrigate IV tubing with NS before and after administration.

Terbutaline

Dosage

- 0.1-10 mcg/kg per minute IV/IO infusion; consider 10 mcg/kg IV/IO load over 5 minutes.

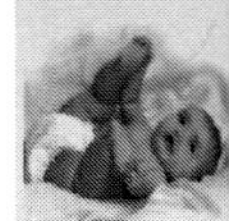

- 10 mcg/kg subcutaneously q10-15 minutes until IV/IO infusion is initiated (max single dose 0.4 mg).

Indications: Asthma (status asthmaticus, hyperkalemia).

Contraindications: Tachyarrhythmias, unstable vasomotor system disorders, hypertension.

Adverse Effects

- **CNS:** Tremors, anxiety, headache, dizziness, stimulation.
- **Cardiovascular:** Palpitations, tachycardia, hypertension, hypotension, arrhythmias, myocardial ischemia.
- **Gastrointestinal:** nausea, vomiting.

Special Nursing Considerations

- Monitor ECG and SpO_2 continuously and blood pressure frequently.
- Like other β_2-adrenergic agonist, terbutaline can lower serum potassium concentrations. The drug should be used cautiously in children with hypokalemia.

Tramadol

Dosage: 1-1.5 mg/kg.

Indications: Relief of moderate to moderately severe pain.

Contraindications: allergy, acute intoxication with alcohol, opioids, psychotropic drugs or other centrally-acting analgesics.

Adverse Effects

- **CNS:** Sedation, dizziness/vertigo. Headache, seizures.
- **Cardiovascular:** Hypotension.
- **Gastrointestinal:** nausea, vomiting.
- **Skin:** sweating, pruritus, rash.

Special Nursing Considerations

- Provide environmental control (temperature, lightning) if sweating, CNS effects occur.
- Administer IV slowly and dilute in normal saline.
- Keep patient in bed if dizziness, vertigo occurs.

Valporic Acid

Dosage: Initial: 10-15 mg/kg/24 hr PO ÷ once daily-TID; Increment: 5-10 mg/kg/24 hr at weekly intervals to max dose of 60 mg/kg/24 hr; Maintenance: 30-60 mg/kg/24 hr ÷ BID-TID.

Indications: Adjunctive therapy in multiple adjunctive types, including absence seizures.

Contraindications: Hepatic disease, significant hepatic dysfunction.

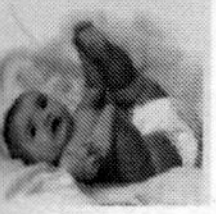

Adverse Effects

- **CNS:** Sedation, tremors, headache, hyperammonic encephalopathy.
- **Gastrointestinal:** nausea, vomiting, indigestion, pancreatitis, hepatic failure, hyperammonia.
- **Hematologic:** Thrombocytopenia, platelet dysfunction, rash.

Special Nursing Considerations

- Administer drug exactly as prescribed.
- Give drug with food if GI upset occurs. Do not administer with carbonated beverages.
- Avoid alcohol, sleep-inducing drugs and over the counter medications.
- Do not stop abruptly, change dose or substitute with other drug.
- Arrange for regular check-up for liver and renal dysfunction.

Vasopressin

Dosage

- **Cardiac arrest:** 0.4-1 unit/kg bolus (max 40 units).
- **Catecholamine-resistant hypotension:** 0.0002-0.002 unit/kg per minute (0.2-2 milliunits/kg per minute) continuous infusion.

  Indications: Cardiac arrest, Catecholamine-resistant hypotension.

  Contra-indications: allergy to vasopressin, chronic nephritis.

Adverse Effects

- **CNS:** Fever, vertigo, water intoxication syndrome.
- **Respiratory:** Bronchial constriction.
- **Cardiovascular:** Arrhythmia, hypertension.
- **Gastrointestinal:** Mesenteric ischemia, nausea, vomiting, abdominal cramps.
- **Genitourinary:** Uterine contraction.
- **Skin:** Urticaria, skin necrosis.

Special Nursing Considerations

- Monitor blood pressure and distal pulses.
- Watch for signs of water intoxication (headaches and drowsiness).
- Use with caution in children with renal insufficiency or hyponatremia/free water overload, asthma or cardiovascular disease.
- Vasoconstriction and tissue necrosis may occur if extravasation is present.

APPENDIX

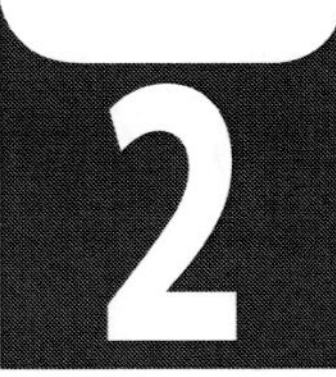

Immunization Schedule

Age	Vaccines
Birth	BCG OPV Zero Hepatitis B-1
6 Weeks	OPV-1 DPT-1 Hepatitis B-2 HIB-1
10 Weeks	OPV-2 DPT-2 HIB-2
14 Weeks	OPV-3 DPT-3 Hepatitis B-3 HIB-3
9 Months	Measles
15-18 Months	OPV-4 DPT-Booster-1 HIB-Booster MMR-1
2 Years	Typhoid
5 Years	OPV-5 DPT Booster-2 MMR-2
10 Years	Combined Tetanus, Diptheria, Pertusis.

(Indian association of paediatrics)

Vaccine which are optional

Age	Vaccines
More than 6 weeks	Pneumococal Conjugate (3 Primary doses at 6, 10, 14 weeks, followed by a booster at 15-18 months)
More than 6 weeks	Rota viral vaccines 2-3 doses (depending on brand) at 4-8 interval
After 15 Months	Varicella Age less than 13 years: 1 dose Age More than 13 years: 2 doses at 4-8 weeks interval
After 18 Months	Hepatitis A (2 doses at 6-12 months interval)

(Indian association of paediatrics)

APPENDIX 3

Normal Values Tables

Normal Values of Vital Signs in Children

Weight	Pulse Rate	Systolic BP	Respiratory Rate	Tidal Volume
3 kg (50-54 cm)	110-160/min	70-90 mm Hg	30-40\min	24 ml
4 kg (55-58 cm)	110-160/min	70-90 mm Hg	30-40\min	24 ml
5 kg (59-61 cm)	110-160/min	70-90 mm Hg	30-40/min	40 ml
6-7 kg (62-68 cm)	110-160/min	70-90 mm Hg	30-40/min	48 ml
8-9 kg (69-75 cm)	100-150/min	80-95 mm Hg	25-35/ min	70 ml
10-11 kg (76-85 cm)	100-150/min	80-85 mm Hg	25-35/ min	85 ml
12-14 kg (86-99 cm)	95-140/min	80-100 mm Hg	25-30 /min	104 ml
15-18 kg (100-113 cm)	95-140/min	80-100 mm Hg	25-30 /min	135 ml
19-23 kg (114-128 cm)	80-120/min	90-110 mm Hg	20-25/min	168 ml
24-29 kg (129-138 cm)	80-120/min	90-110 mm Hg	20-25/min	215 ml
30-36 kg (139-148 cm)	80-120/min	90-110 mm Hg	20-25/min	265 ml

Common Sizes of Resuscitation Equipment

Weight	ETT size uncuffed	ETT Length	Laryngoscope
3 kg (50-54 cm)	3.5	9-9.5 cm	1 S
4 kg (55-58 cm)	3.5	9.5-10cm	1 S
5 kg (59-61 cm)	3.5	10-10.5 cm	1 S
6-7 kg (62-68 cm)	3.5	10.5-11cm	1 S
8-9 kg (69-75 cm)	3.5	10.5-11cm	1 S
10-11 kg (76-85 cm)	4	11-12 cm	1 S
12-14 kg (86-99 cm)	4.5	13.5 cm	2 S
15-18 kg (100-113 cm)	5	14-15 cm	2 S
19-23 kg (114-128 cm)	5.5	16.5 cm	2 S or C
24-29 kg (129-138 cm)	6.0	17-18 cm	2 S or C
30-36 kg (139-148 cm)	6.5	18.5 – 19.5	3 S or C

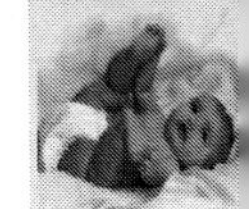

Common Sizes of Various Tubes

Weight	Suction Catheter	NG tube	Chest tube	Urinary Cath.
3 kg (50-54 cm)	8 F	5-8 F	10-12 F	5-6 F
4 kg (55-58 cm)	8 F	5-8 F	10-12 F	5-6 F
5 kg (59-61 cm)	8 F	5-8 F	10-12 F	5-6 F
6-7 kg (62-68 cm)	8 F	5-8 F	10-12 F	5-6 F
8-9 kg (69-75 cm)	8 F	5-8 F	10-12 F	8 F
10-11 kg (76-85 cm)	10 F	8-10 F	16-20 F	8-10 F
12-14 kg (86-99 cm)	10 F	10 F	20-24 F	10 F
15-18 kg (100-113cm)	10 F	10 F	20-24 F	10-12 F
19-23 kg (114-128 cm)	10 F	12-14 F	24-32 F	10-12 F
24-29 kg (129-138 cm)	10 F	14-18 F	28-32 F	12 F
30-36 kg (139-148 cm)	10-12 F	16-18 F	32- 38 F	12 F